GASTROENTEROLOGY AND HEPATOLOGY

The Comprehensive Visual Reference

GASTROENTEROLOGY AND HEPATOLOGY

The Comprehensive Visual Reference

series editor
Mark Feldman, MD

Southland Professor and Vice Chairman
Department of Internal Medicine
University of Texas Southwestern
  Medical Center at Dallas

Chief, Medical Service
Veterans Affairs Medical Center
Dallas, Texas

volume 8
Pancreas

volume editor
Phillip P. Toskes, MD

Professor and Chairman
Department of Medicine
University of Florida College of Medicine
Gainsville, Florida

With 13 contributors

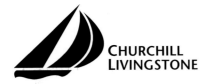

**CHURCHILL
LIVINGSTONE**

Developed by Current Medicine, Inc.
Philadelphia

Current Medicine, Inc.

400 Market Street
Suite 700
Philadelphia, PA 19106

Managing Editor	*Lori J. Bainbridge*
Development Editors	*Ira D. Smiley and Raymond Lukens*
Editorial Assistant	*Scott Thomas Hurd*
Art Director	*Paul Fennessy*
Design and Layout	*Robert LeBrun*
Illustration Director	*Ann Saydlowski*
Illustrators	*Liz Carrozza, Larry Ward, Lisa Weischedel, and Debra Wertz*
Typesetting	*Ryan Walsh*
Production	*Lori Holland and Sally Nicholson*
Indexer	*Maria Coughlin*

Pancreas /Phillip P. Toskes, volume editor.
        p. cm. — (Gastroenterology and hepatology: v. 8)
    Includes bibliographical references and index.
    ISBN 0-443-07862-9
    1. Pancreas—Diseases—Atlases. 2. Pancreas—Atlases.
I. Toskes, Phillip P. (Phillip Paul), 1940- .
II. Series.
    [DNLM: 1. Pancreatic Diseases—atlases. 2. Pancreas—surgery—atlases. 1998
A-754 v.8 / WI 17 G257 1998 v. 8]
RC857.P283 1998
616.3'7—dc21
DNLM/DLC
for Library of Congress   98-5985
                                                                            CIP

Library of Congress Cataloging-in-Publication Data
ISBN 0-443-07862-9

Printed in Singapore by Imago Productions (FE) Pte Ltd.

10 9 8 7 6 5 4 3 2 1

Although every effort has been made to ensure that drug doses and other information are presented accurately in this publication, the ultimate responsibility rests with the prescribing physician. Neither the publishers nor the authors can be held responsible for errors or for any consequences arising from the use of information contained herein. Products mentioned in this publication should be used in accordance with the prescribing information prepared by the manufacturers. No claims or endorsements are made for any drug or compound at present under clinical investigation.

DISTRIBUTED WORLDWIDE BY CHURCHILL LIVINGSTONE, INC.

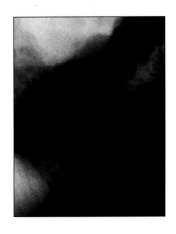

Series Preface

In recent years dramatic developments in the practice of gastro-enterology have unfolded, and the specialty has become, more than ever, a visual discipline. Advances in endoscopy, radiology, or a combination of the two, such as endoscopic retrograde cholangiopancreatography and endoscopic ultrasonography, have occurred in the past 2 decades. Because of advanced imaging technology, a gastroenterologist, like a dermatologist, is often able to directly view the pathology of a patient's organs. Moreover, practicing gastroenterologists and hepatologists can frequently diagnose disease from biopsy samples examined microscopically, often aided by an increasing number of special staining techniques. As a result of these advances, gastroenterology has grown as rapidly as any subspecialty of internal medicine.

Gastroenterology and Hepatology: The Comprehensive Visual Reference is an ambitious 8-volume collection of images that pictorially displays the gastrointestinal tract, liver, biliary tree, and pancreas in health and disease, both in children and adults. The series is comprised of 89 chapters containing nearly 4000 images accompanied by legends. The images in this collection include not only traditional photographs but also charts, tables, drawings, algorithms, and diagrams, making this collection much more than an atlas in the conventional sense. Chapters are authored by experts selected by one of the eight volume editors, who carefully reviewed each chapter within their volume.

Disorders of the gastrointestinal tract, liver, biliary tree, and pancreas are common in children and adults. *Helicobacter pylori* gastritis is the most frequent bacterial infection of humans and is a risk factor for peptic ulcer disease and gastric malignancies. Colorectal carcinoma is the second leading cause of cancer mortality in the United States, with nearly 60,000 deaths in 1990. Pancreatic cancer resulted in an additional 25,000 deaths. Liver disease is also an important cause of morbidity and mortality, with more that 25,000 deaths from cirrhosis alone in 1990. Gallstone disease is also common in our society, with increasing reliance on laparoscopic cholecystectomy in symptomatic individuals. Inflammatory bowel diseases (ulcerative colitis, Crohn's disease) are also widespread in all segments of the population; their causes still elude us.

The past few decades have also witnessed striking advances in the therapy of gastrointestinal disorders. Examples include "cure" of peptic ulcer disease by eradicating *H. pylori* with antimicrobial agents, healing of erosive esophagitis with proton pump inhibitor drugs, remission of chronic viral hepatitis B or C with interferon-α2b, and hepatic transplantation for patients with fulminant hepatic failure or end-stage liver disease. Therapeutic endoscopic techniques have proliferated that ameliorate the need for surgical procedures. Endoscopic advances include placement of peroral endoscopic gastrostomy tubes for nutritional support, insertion of stents in the bile duct or esophagus to relieve malignant obstruction, and the use of injection therapy, thermal coagulation, or laser therapy to treat bleeding ulcers and other lesions, including tumors. *Gastroenterology and Hepatology: The Comprehensive Visual Reference* will cover these advances and many others in the field of gastroenterology.

I wish to thank a number of people for their contributions to this series. The dedication and expertise of the other volume editors—Willis Maddrey, Rick Boland, Paul Hyman, Nick LaRusso, Roy Orlando, Larry Schiller, and Phil Toskes—was critical and most appreciated. The nearly 100 contributing authors were both creative and generous with their time and teaching materials. And special thanks to Abe Krieger, President of Current Medicine, for recruiting me for this unique project, and to his talented associates at Current Medicine.

The images contained in this 8-volume collection are available in print as well as in slide format, and the series is soon being formatted for CD-ROM use. All of us who have participated in this ambitious project hope that each of the 8 volumes, as well as the entire collection, will be useful to physicians and health professionals throughout the world involved in the diagnosis and treatment of patients of all ages who suffer from gastrointestinal disorders.

Mark Feldman, MD

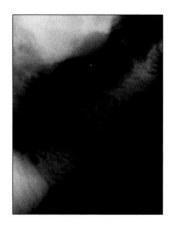

Volume Preface

The pancreas is a remarkable organ that plays a pivotal role in both digestion and metabolism of nutrients. Although the pathogenesis of both acute and chronic pancreatitis remains to be fully defined, significant progress has been made in several areas of pancreatic physiology and pathophysiology in the past several years. The contributors to the 10 chapters in this volume are all acknowledged experts in the field of pancreatic function and dysfunction.

David C. Whitcomb's chapter on "Neurohormonal Control of the Pancreas" integrates old and new information to present a unified model. The focus is on physiological mechanisms related to acid neutralization and protein digestion. Major functions of the pancreas include secretion of bicarbonate into the duodenum to neutralize the acid chyme exiting the stomach; secretion of digestive enzymes into the duodenum where the breakdown of complex proteins, carbohydrates, lipids, and nucleic acids occurs; and secretion of islet cell hormones into the circulation to control systemic metabolism of nutrients after absorption. The role of the nervous system, the major stimulatory hormones (cholecystokinin [CCK] and secretin), and the inhibitory hormones (pancreatic polypeptide, peptide YY, and somatostatin) are emphasized in the context of normal pancreatic function.

Recent studies demonstrate, both in animals and humans, that CCK acts through the cholinergic pathways to mediate pancreatic secretion of enzymes and bicarbonate. In addition, depending on the stimulants, it appears that the release of CCK from the small intestine may be modulated by cholinergic input. Secretin, the other main hormone that controls pancreatic secretion, appears to be regulated by a capsaicin-sensitive vagal afferent mechanism. Together these findings modify greatly our understanding of the mechanisms of action of CCK and secretin on pancreatic exocrine secretion.

James H. Grendell notes that acute pancreatitis, chronic pancreatitis, and pancreatic cancer are common diseases worldwide. Although the etiologies and risk factors for these disorders can often be identified, the pathogenesis of pancreatitis and pancreatic cancer is not well understood. His chapter reviews current theories of pathogenesis of pancreatic disease, indicating areas in which therapeutic modifications can be made. The activation of the cytokine cascade appears to play an important role in the evolution of the complications of acute pancreatitis. The role of nitrous oxide in reducing the severity of acute pancreatitis has also been an area of intense interest. Although it was once thought that our understanding of the pathogenesis of chronic pancreatitis (at least alcohol-induced chronic pancreatitis) was firm, now those concepts have been challenged. Dr. Grendell discusses several possible therapies for the causation of chronic

pancreatitis. Pancreatic cancer is a devastating disease. New knowledge is needed in our understanding of risk factors, pathogenesis, and therapy. A greater understanding of the cell biology factors regulating growth and differentiation in the pancreas and in the molecular biology of tumor genesis may lead to important advances in our understanding of the pathogenesis of this cancer and to breakthroughs in gene therapy and therapy directed at inhibiting cell growth.

William Steinberg describes acute pancreatitis as a common disorder whose pathogenesis remains obscure. On a worldwide basis, gallstones are the leading etiologic cause, followed by alcoholism. A significant number of people with acute pancreatitis have no detectable cause. The diagnosis of acute pancreatitis is usually made clinically using blood levels of enzymes, with lipase being more sensitive and specific than amylase. Sonography is the best imaging technique for diagnosing gallstone pancreatitis; although during the acute attack, its sensitivity is only 70% to 80%. Computed tomography (CT) is reserved for later use to determine if pancreatic necrosis is present, to confirm the diagnosis, to look for tumors as an unusual cause of pancreatitis, and to monitor fluid collections during the second week of hospitalization.

Although the Ranson and APACHE criteria are commonly used in the United States to monitor the severity of pancreatitis, these scoring systems have shortcomings. The search continues for a single test to determine which patients will have a stormy course. Although acute pancreatitis tends to be a mild disease, complications can occur in up to 25% of patients, with a mortality rate of nearly 10%. Treatment has been largely conservative management, but certain specific therapies have proved promising. Emergency endoscopic retrograde cholangiopancreatography in patients with suspected gallstone pancreatitis and removal of stones from the common duct may improve the prognosis of severe pancreatitis and does not seem to worsen mild pancreatitis. The antimicrobial drug imipenem given soon after admission reduces pancreatic and nonpancreatic infection in severe necrotizing pancreatitis. The role of surgical therapy in severe pancreatitis needs to be redefined.

Chris Forsmark and Phillip P. Toskes describe the value of classifying chronic pancreatitis into big-duct and small-duct disease. There are many causes of pancreatitis, but all ultimately lead to irreversible morphological damage to the pancreas. However, treatment can reduce the cardinal complications of chronic pancreatitis (abdominal pain, steatorrhea, and diabetes mellitus). Although long-term alcohol abuse is the most common cause, other important causes include obstruction of the main pancreatic duct, hyperlipidemia, and idiopathic forms, which may account for up to 25% of cases.

The natural history of chronic pancreatitis is one of progressive destruction of the gland occurring over 10 to 20 years, but the natural histories of alcoholic and idiopathic chronic pancreatitis are quite different. Patients with chronic pancreatitis present to the clinician because of abdominal pain, signs or symptoms of maldigestion, or both. The diagnosis of chronic pancreatitis is relatively easy in patients with severe, advanced disease but very difficult in patients who have small-duct disease and no signs of maldigestion.

Treatment of the patient begins with the recognition that chronic pancreatitis may be present and that some of the complications (*eg*, duodenal or binary obstruction or a symptomatic pseudocyst) require specific therapy. Cessation of alcohol consumption, treatment of malnutrition and steatorrhea, and therapy with analgesics are useful. Medical therapy for chronic pain may also include agents that reduce excessive feedback stimulation of the pancreas and, in particular, non–enteric-coated pancreatic enzymes. Patients with big-duct disease who fail medical therapy are candidates for surgical duct decompression or treatment with octreotide.

Stephen B. Vogel presents the surgical therapy for chronic pancreatitis. The decision to operate, Dr. Vogel tells us, is often clear and based on alleviation of pain, elimination of recurrent attacks of pain, and treating pancreatic pseudocysts independently of complications occurring after their formation. The management of pancreatic pseudocysts has become more conservative and the use of high-resolution CT allows more appropriate management of these pseudocysts. The mainstay of surgical treatment of chronic pancreatitis is internal pancreatic duct drainage in patients with moderately to widely dilated pancreatic ductal systems. Although such an operation often relieves the unremitting pain in these unfortunate patients, it is controversial as to whether or not ductal decompression preserves exocrine and endocrine function. Dr. Vogel also covers special circumstances related to chronic pancreatitis in which advances have been made in both diagnosis and treatment, including pancreatic ascites, infection, trauma, and hereditary pancreatitis.

Glen A. Lehman contributes a thorough review of developmental anomalies of the pancreas.

These anomalies are, by definition, present at birth but are not commonly suspected or detected until adulthood. In reality, most developmental anomalies and variances of the pancreas are of no clinical significance and are detected coincidentally at endoscopy, surgery, or autopsy. In selected settings, these alterations have clinical consequences. Dr. Lehman's chapter focuses mostly on adult patients in these settings. Although significant congenital anomalies of the pancreas presenting in childhood are generally detected by CT scans or other studies, endoscopic detection and management are being increasingly used.

Mark T. Toyama, Ann M. Kusske, and Howard A. Reber discuss the deadliness of pancreatic cancer and its increasing frequency. It is the fourth most common cause of death from cancer. Almost 95% of all patients afflicted with this disease eventually die. African Americans in the United States have one of the highest risks for pancreatic cancer in the world. Other than cigarette smoking, few definitive risk factors for pancreatic cancer have been identified. Most pancreatic cancers are adenocarcinomas that originate from the pancreatic main duct. The best hope to cure pancreatic cancer depends on an early diagnosis, which at present cannot be accomplished.. Pancreatic carcinoma often presents nonspecifically. Biochemical markers used as potential aids in the diagnosis of this disease are discussed. The most widely used is CA19-9, which correlates with tumor burden.

The use of both percutaneous and endoscopic stents has eliminated the need for surgery in some patients with pancreatic cancer. The standard operative treatment for resectable pancreatic cancer is pancreaticoduodenectomy. The morbidity and mortality rates of this operation have improved dramatically, 15% and less than 5%, respectively. However, the long-term survival rate is only about 10%. Biliary intestinal bypass can provide excellent palliation to patients with unresectable pancreatic cancer. Medical options in the treatment of pancreatic cancer are limited, and survival is usually less than 1 year. Treatment options include radiotherapy, chemotherapy, hormonal therapy, immunotherapy, and a combination of these treatments with or without surgery. Pancreatic cancer patients with the best chance of survival are those in whom the cancer is detected early and who undergo a curative resection.

Rodney V. Pozderac and Thomas M. O'Dorisio discuss the rationale and application of radioligand imaging in pancreatic disorders. Octreotide has been successfully radiolabeled and used to visualize pancreatic neuroendocrine tumors. The authors describe their extensive experience at Ohio State University Medical Center using tyrosinated somatostatin analogs. They have been able to localize somatostatin-receptive carcinoid tumors and such neuroendocrine tumors as gastrinoma, glucagonoma, and neuroblastoma—the childhood neuroendocrine tumor. In many instances, a positive, radiolabeled somatostatin scintigraphy predicts a favorable response to octreotide therapy.

Peter R. Durie contributes a comprehensive description of pancreatic disorders in children. While cystic fibrosis is the most important childhood pancreatic disorder, other entities may mimic cystic fibrosis and must be considered. The approach to the child with pancreatic disease may be similar to that of the adult, but at times the management in the child may be unique. Approximately 80% of children with cystic fibrosis may develop severe maldigestion and, at a later age, may present themselves to adult gastroenterologists for management. Management of the pulmonary complications in cystic fibrosis has improved survival remarkably, and more afflicted children live to be adults.

David C. Whitcomb presents an exciting contribution on hereditary pancreatitis that may provide fundamental insights into the cause of both acute and chronic pancreatitis due to other etiologies. Hereditary pancreatitis is a rare, chronic, idiopathic inflammatory disorder that affects multiple family members over two or more generations. Inheritance occurs as an autosomal trait with variable expression. Using genetic linkage analysis and positional cloning, a mutation causing hereditary pancreatitis was discovered in the cationic trypsinogen gene. This mutant form of trypsin is resistant to intrapancreatic inactivation, which leads to typical acute and chronic pancreatitis and predisposes to pancreatic cancer. The discovery of this mutation provides key insights into all major forms of pancreatitis and pancreatic diseases.

I want to personally express my sincere gratitude for the fine contributions made to this volume by all of the participants named above. Despite the fact that more information is needed about pancreatic physiology and pathophysiology, the enclosed chapters offer an impressive account of new developments to enhance our understanding of pancreatic function and dysfunction and to lead to potential new therapies.

Phillip P. Toskes, MD

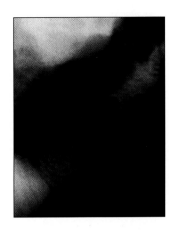

Contributors

Peter R. Durie, BsC, MD, FRCPC
Head, Division of Gastroenterology and Nutrition
The Hospital for Sick Children
Toronto, Ontario, Canada

Christopher E. Forsmark, MD
Associate Professor
Department of Medicine
University of Florida College of Medicine
Shands Hospital at the University of Florida
Gainesville, Florida

James H. Grendell, MD
Professor
Department of Medicine
Cornell University Medical College
Chief, Division of Digestive Diseases
New York Hospital-Cornell Medical Center
New York, New York

Amy M. Kusske, MD
Resident
Department of Surgery
University of California, Los Angeles, School of Medicine
Los Angeles, California

Glen A. Lehman, MD
Professor of Medicine
Department of Radiology and Medicine
Indiana School of Medicine;
Indiana University Medical Center
Indianapolis, Indiana

Thomas M. O'Dorisio, MD
Professor of Medicine
The Ohio State University College of Medicine
The Ohio State University Medical Center
Columbus, Ohio

Rodney V. Pozderac, MD
Clinical Associate Professor
Department of Radiology
Ohio State University
The Ohio State University Medical Center
Columbus, Ohio

Howard A. Reber, MD
Professor
Department of Surgery
University of California, Los Angeles, School of Medicine
Los Angeles, California

William M. Steinberg, MD
Professor
Department of Medicine
George Washington University School of Medicine and Health
    Sciences
Washington, DC

Phillip P. Toskes, MD
Professor and Chairman
Department of Medicine
University of Florida College of Medicine
Gainesville, Florida

Mark T. Toyama, MD
Resident
Department of Surgery
University of California, Los Angeles, School of Medicine
Los Angeles, California

Stephen B. Vogel, MD
Professor
Department of Surgery
University of Florida College of Medicine
Shands Hospital
Gainesville, Florida

David C. Whitcomb, MD
Associate Professor
Department of Medicine
University of Pittsburgh School of Medicine
University of Pittsburgh Medical Center
Pittsburgh VA Health Care System
Pittsburgh, Pennsylvania

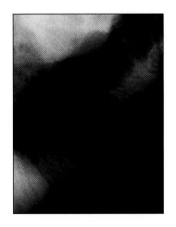

Contents

Chapter 9
Cystic Fibrosis
PETER R. DURIE

Chapter 10
Hereditary Pancreatitis
DAVID C. WHITCOMB

Index

Chapter 1

Neurohormonal Control of the Pancreas

DAVID C. WHITCOMB

The pancreas is a vital organ that plays a central role in digestion and in the metabolism of nutrients. Major functions of the pancreas include secretion of bicarbonate into the duodenum to neutralize the acid chyme exiting the stomach; secretion of digestive enzymes into the duodenum for the breakdown of complex proteins, carbohydrates, lipids, and nucleic acids; and secretion of islet cell hormones into the circulation to control systemic metabolism of nutrients after absorption.

The diverse and irregular dietary practices of animals require a versatile mechanism to control pancreatic function. Careful observation of the pattern of pancreatic secretion reveals initiation of pancreatic secretion with the sight and smell of food (the cephalic phase), further stimulation of secretion with gastric distention (gastric phase), and the greatest degree of secretion corresponding to the delivery of undigested nutrients into the duodenum (intestinal phase). The additional observation that the volume and content of pancreatic secretion are governed by the size and nutritional content of a meal further suggests a well-designed control system.

The common view of pancreatic secretory control involves the release of a hormone bolus by a meal that circulates to the pancreas and causes it to secrete "a meal's worth" of bicarbonate and enzymes. In humans, pancreatic secretion is actually controlled by more complex and integrated neurohormonal reflexes, which include feedback controls. Thus, bicarbonate secretion is closely tied to the immediate duodenal hydrogen-ion concentration; pancreatic enzyme secretion is tied to the activity of the duodenal proteolytic enzymes. Pancreatic secretion is further modified by central and peripheral factors related to the anticipation and progression of digestion and absorption.

Many of the mechanisms involved in the control of pancreatic exocrine secretion have recently been clarified. This chapter integrates old and new information to present a unified model of explaining the neurohormonal control of the pancreas. The focus is on physiologic mechanisms related to acid neutralization and protein digestion. The role of the nervous system, the major stimulatory hormones (cholecystokinin and secretin), and the inhibitory hormones (pancreatic polypeptide, peptide YY, and somatostatin) are emphasized in the context of normal pancreatic function.

■ HISTORICAL BACKGROUND

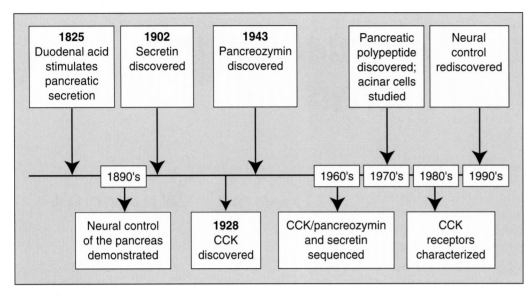

FIGURE 1-1.

Major discoveries in pancreatic exocrine physiology. Investigation of the mechanism controlling pancreatic secretion began in 1825, when it was determined that acidification of the upper gastrointestinal tract increased the flow of pancreatic juice. Ivan Petrovich Pavlov, the great Russian physiologist, and his students used innovative experiments during the last half of the 19th century to establish and define the role of the central nervous system in controlling the pancreas. The field of endocrinology was born in 1902 with the discovery by Bayliss and Starling [1] of the hormone *secretin*. Between 1902 and 1966 the importance of hormones was established, culminating in the isolation and sequencing of secretin and cholecystokinin (CCK). Receptor identification and localization further advanced our understanding of pancreatic physiology during the 1980s. Among these important findings was the discovery of the pancreatic enzyme-stimulating CCK-A receptors in the brain and afferent vagal fibers, and also the determination that neither the CCK-A receptor, nor its mRNA, is present in human acinar cells. These recent discoveries suggest that the major hormone mechanisms are indirect and that there is an important interplay between hormonal and neural mechanisms that control the pancreas.

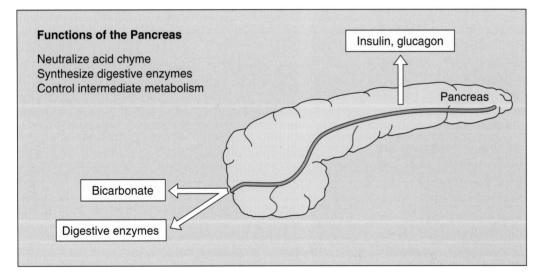

Functions of the Pancreas

Neutralize acid chyme
Synthesize digestive enzymes
Control intermediate metabolism

Insulin, glucagon

Pancreas

Bicarbonate

Digestive enzymes

FIGURE 1-2.

Physiologic function of the pancreas. The human pancreas has three general functions: (1) neutralizing the acid chyme entering the duodenum from the stomach; (2) synthesis and secretion of digestive enzymes after a meal; and (3) systemic release of hormones that modulate metabolism of carbohydrates, proteins, and lipids.

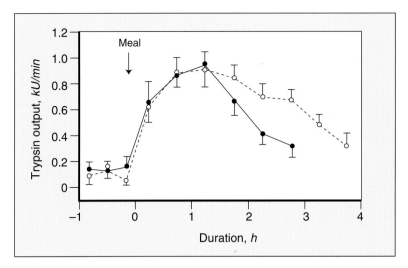

FIGURE 1-3.

Pancreatic exocrine secretion is controlled by integrated neural and hormonal mechanisms. In the interdigestive period the pancreas is generally quiescent. With the sight and smell of food, however, the pancreas becomes one of the most metabolically active organs in the body. The secretory response of the pancreas corresponds to size, consistency, and nutritional content of a meal. The responsiveness of the pancreas to variations in diet suggests the existence of a well-defined control system. This figure illustrates the prolongation of trypsin secretion with a solid meal compared with a liquid meal. Several recent discoveries have caused physicians and scientists to question classical models explaining the stimulation of pancreatic secretion and to introduce new, integrated models of neurohormonal control. (*Adapted from* Malagelada [2]; with permission.)

ANATOMY OF THE PANCREATIC CONTROL SYSTEM

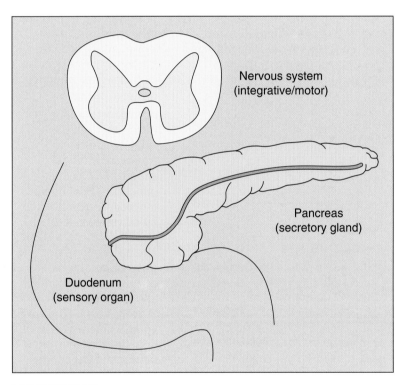

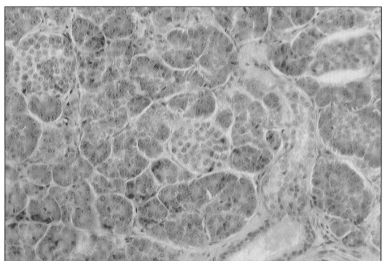

FIGURE 1-4.

Pancreatic control system. Most pancreatic exocrine secretion is controlled through three systems. The duodenum and gastrointestinal tract act as the primary sensory organs for pancreatic function; the sensory information is relayed through nervous and hormonal mechanisms. The nervous system includes portions of the central nervous system, sensory and motor divisions of the autonomic nervous system, and an intrapancreatic nervous system. The nervous system is critical for integration of sensory and hormonal information and stimulation of pancreatic secretion. The pancreas is the glandular structure wherein all stimulatory pathways converge on the ductal and acinar cells.

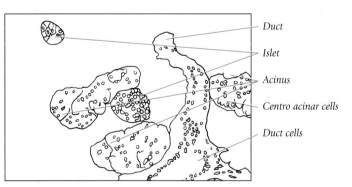

FIGURE 1-5.

Overview of the pancreatic gland. The pancreatic gland contains three major types of cells. The *duct* cells make up about 10% of the pancreas and secrete solutions rich in bicarbonate. The *acinar* cells comprise over 80% of the pancreas and they synthesize and secrete pancreatic enzymes. The *islet* cells make up about 10% of the pancreas and form the endocrine portion of the pancreas. The four major types of islet cells secrete the hormones insulin, glucagon, somatostatin, and pancreatic polypeptide.

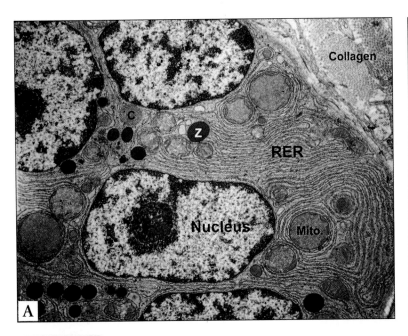

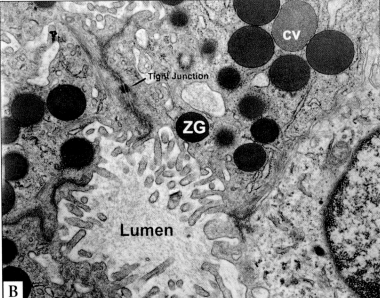

A–B, Electron micrographs of pancreatic acinar cells. The basolateral-sided pancreatic acinar cells (**panel A**) have an extensive network of rough endoplasmic reticulum (RER) for the synthesis of pancreatic digestive enzymes (zymogens). After syntenesis the zymogens move to the golgi, where they are sorted from other cellular proteins packaged into condensing vacules (cv). The cv condense to become zymogen granules (Z and ZG) and move to the apical side of the acinar cell (**panel B**). Upon stimulation, the contents of the ZGs empty into the lumen of the acinus and begin moving through the pancreatic ducts toward the intestinal lumen. Mito—mitochondria.

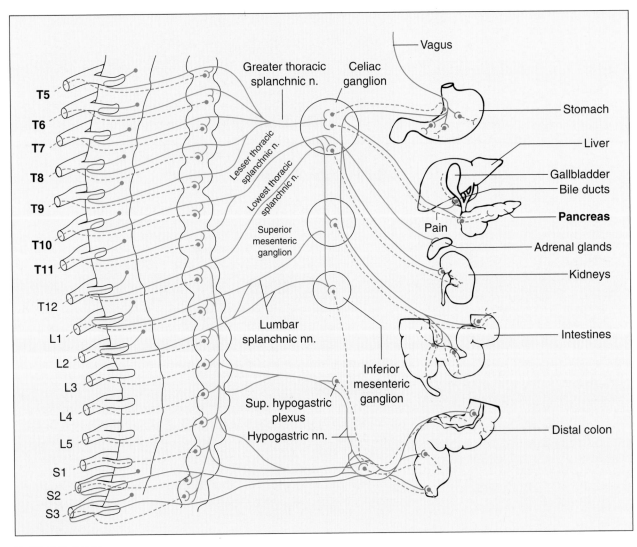

Overview of the neural innervation of the pancreas. The pancreas is innervated by the sympathetic, para-sympathetic, and enteric nervous systems. The sympathetic input to the pancreas arises in the spinal cord at primarily from T5–T9, travels through the splanchnic nerves, through the celiac ganglia, and to the pancreas. These nerves innervate intrapancreatic blood vessels and ganglia, and also carry pain fibers. The parasympathetic innervation travels through the vagus nerve and includes motor and sensory fibers. The pancreas also receives input directly from myenteric neurons of the enteric nervous systems. Finally, the pancreas contains a network of nerves and ganglia encompassing blood vessels, acinar cells, and islets. Major neurotransmitters responsible for pancreatic exocrine secretion include acetylcholine, vasoactive intestinal peptide, gastrin-releasing peptide, and others. Integration of the neural and hormonal systems constitutes the pancreatic control system. (*Adapted from Netter [2a]; with permission.*)

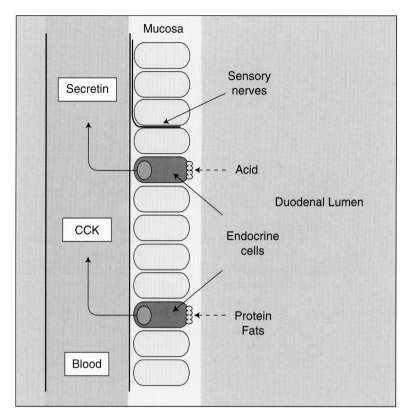

Figure 1-8.

Overview of the duodenum. The duodenum is the most important sensory organ involved in pancreatic secretion, and is the site where the meal and pancreatic exocrine secretions meet. The duodenal mucosa contains endocrine cells, which release secretin in response to luminal acid, and cholecystokinin (CCK) in response to proteins or fats. The duodenum is also rich in sensory (afferent) vagal nerve fibers that respond to changes in pH, amino acids, lipids, and express receptors for CCK and secretin.

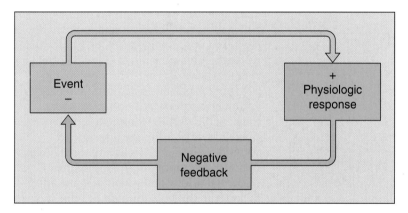

Figure 1-9.

Feedback: control mechanisms. The pancreas uses the basic physiologic principle of feedback inhibition to facilitate accurate delivery of bicarbonate, proteolytic enzymes, and metabolic hormones. The basic components of a feedback control system are illustrated. An "event" (*eg*, acid in the duodenum) serves as a stimulus for a physiologic response (*eg*, secretion of bicarbonate). The response serves to reverse or inhibit the event that stimulates the "physiologic response." The response continues until the stimulus is eliminated. Thus, the response is tightly linked to the event and homeostasis is maintained.

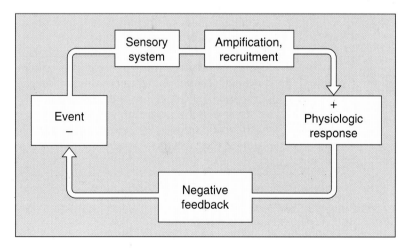

Figure 1-10.

Sensation and amplification. For a feedback system to work under physiologic conditions, the simple feedback system requires several additional components. These include a sensory system (*eg*, in the duodenum) to detect the event and an amplification system to effect an adequate response. If the stimulus is great, parallel systems may also be activated. Typical feedback systems also include mechanisms that potentiate or inhibit the magnitude of the response.

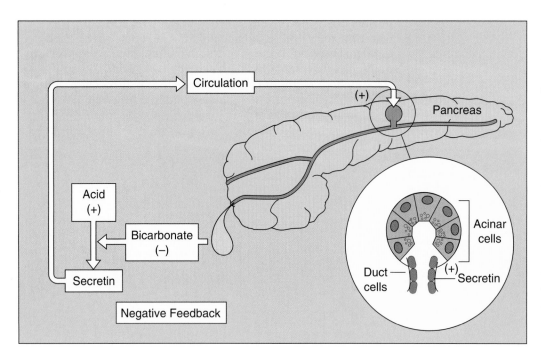

FIGURE 1-11.

Neurohormonal control of pancreatic bicarbonate secretion. The pancreas plays a major role in neutralizing acidic chyme. The event, or stimulus, is the presence of duodenal acid, and the physiologic response is the pancreatic duct cells' secretion of bicarbonate secretion, which enters into the duodenum and neutralizes the duodenal acid. The mechanism of sensation, amplification, and modulation is not fully understood, but the hormone secretin plays a central role. Thus, when the duodenum becomes acidic, secretin is released from endocrine cells in the duodenal mucosa, where it enters the blood stream. Pancreatic duct cells respond by secretion of bicarbonate-rich fluid until the duodenal pH is neutral, thus eliminating the stimulus and completing a negative feedback loop.

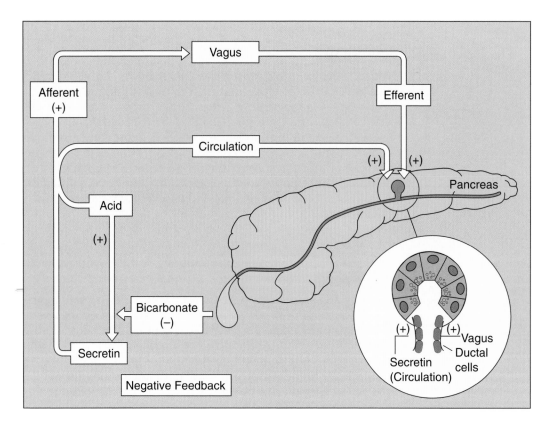

FIGURE 1-12.

The vagus and bicarbonate secretion. The parasympathetic nervous system probably plays a major role in pancreatic bicarbonate secretion. This view is based on the observation that stimulation of the vagal trunk produces pancreatic bicarbonate secretions approaching peak secretion seen after a meal, and that acute transection of the vagus markedly diminishes the response to secretin. The afferent (sensory) vagal fibers may also be important in sensing the duodenal acidity and amplifying the effect of secretin, possibly through secretin receptors on afferent vagal fibers. This view is also supported by studies in the rat that demonstrate blockade of the effects of "physiologic" plasma concentrations of secretin with selective elimination of the afferent vagal fibers by the sensory neurotoxin capsaicin. As the dose of secretin increases, however, a larger fraction of the response is independent of the vagus nerve, suggesting recruitment of other mechanisms, including direct stimulation of ductal cells.

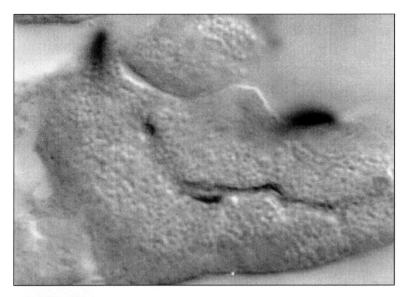

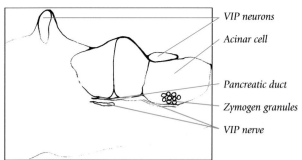

FIGURE 1-13.

Other factors stimulate bicarbonate secretion from the pancreas. A brisk increase in pancreatic fluid secretion, which is rich in bicarbonate, follows electrical stimulation of the vagus nerve in most species. The primary neurotransmitters involved in stimulating bicarbonate release are acetylcholine and vasoactive intestinal peptide (VIP) and related peptides. This photomicrograph of a pancreatic lobule from the rat (note the zymogen granules in the apical end of the acinar cells) reveals a VIP- immunoreactive neuron with axons surrounding an intralobular duct. The close relationship between VIP-positive nerves and the ducts has also been demonstrated in the pig [3]. Although secretin plays a central and early role in stimulating bicarbonate secretion, several neurohormonal systems converge on the final pathway to the ductal cells. These features allow for amplification or inhibition of secretin's effects, depending in part on other important factors related to the meal. Furthermore, these features may provide alternative pathways to the ductal cells as an adaptive mechanism if disease or injury damages the predominant pathway.

Digestion of proteins: The role of cholecystokinin

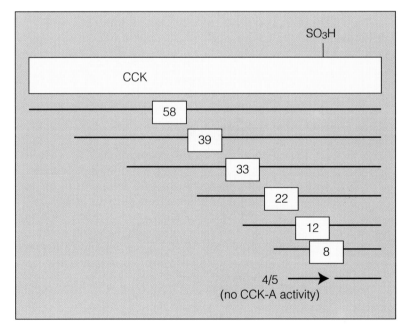

FIGURE 1-14.

Cholecystokinin (CCK) is the most important hormone that influences pancreatic secretion. The humoral substance that caused pancreatic enzyme secretion was identified in duodenal mucosa in 1943 by Harper and Raper [4] and named pancreozymin (PZ). Isolation and sequencing of this factor in 1966 by Mutt and Jorpes [5] proved that PZ and CCK represented two physiological actions of the same molecule. Because this peptide was first recognized and named by Ivy and Oldburg in 1928 [6], only the name cholecystokinin is now used.

CCK is a single-chain peptide that is found in lengths of 4, 5, 8, 12, 22, 33, 39, and 58 amino acids. The biologic activity is located in the common carboxy-terminal end, which contains a sulfated tyrosine at position 7 (note the SO_3H in the figure). The sulfate makes CCK 1000 times more potent than nonsulfated CCK at the CCK-A receptor (*A* indicates alimentary tract), which stimulates pancreatic exocrine secretion. CCK 4 and 5 are in highest concentrations in the brain and act potently on the CCK-B receptor (*B* indicates brain). They have decreased activity on the CCK-A receptor because the sulfated tyrosine is absent.

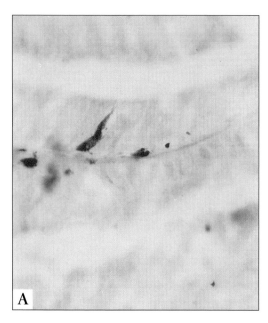

A

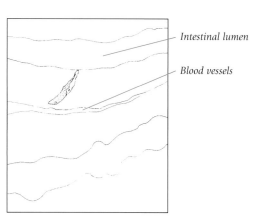

Intestinal lumen

Blood vessels

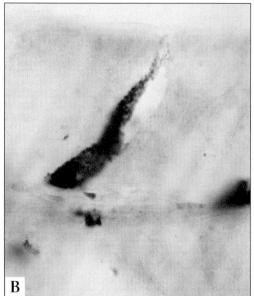

B

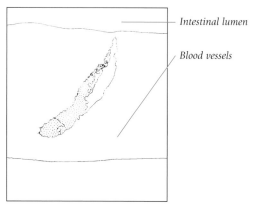

Intestinal lumen

Blood vessels

FIGURE 1-15.

Origin of cholecystokinin (CCK). Synthesis of CCK occurs in endocrine cells of the intestine, neurons of the brain, and in the enteric and pancreatic nervous systems. CCK endocrine cells (**panel A** and **panel B**) are located in the mucosa of the proximal small intestine. The apical ends of the neuroendocrine cells are in direct contact with the intestinal lumen. CCK is released at the basal end near the blood vessels of the intestinal villi. (Note the heavy CCK-immunohistochemical staining at the basal end of the CCK cell.) CCK-synthesizing nerves are found throughout the small and large intestines. CCK-containing neurons are also found in the pancreas; however, these fibers extend to intrapancreatic ganglia and islets rather than to the acinar cells.

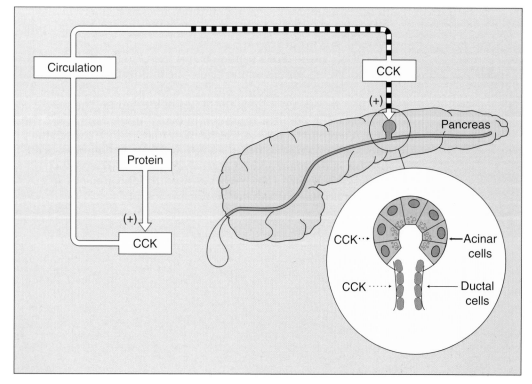

Circulation

CCK

(+)

Pancreas

Protein

(+)

CCK

CCK ·····> Acinar cells

CCK ·····> Ductal cells

FIGURE 1-16.

Actions of cholecystokinin (CCK). CCK is released by a meal, stimulates pancreatic enzyme secretion, and augments bicarbonate secretion. Blocking the effects of CCK with specific CCK-A receptor blockers inhibits pancreatic enzyme secretion by more than 80%, suggesting that CCK plays a major role in stimulating pancreatic secretion.

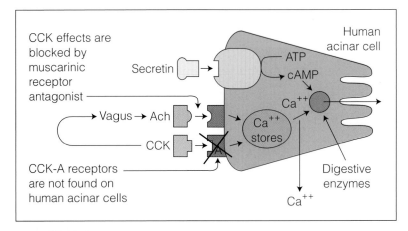

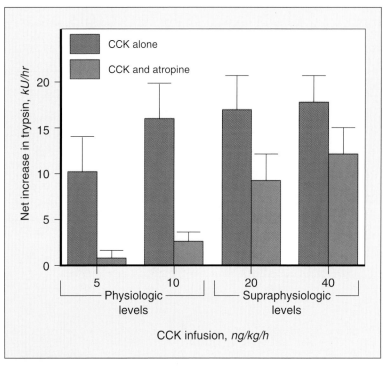

FIGURE 1-17.

Neurohormonal control of digestive enzyme secretion. Understanding of the mechanisms controlling pancreatic enzyme secretion has been revolutionized during the 1990s. Previous models envisioned the release of cholecystokinin (CCK) from the duodenum into the bloodstream, which circulated to the pancreatic acinar cells in which CCK bound to CCK receptors, and thus triggered pancreatic secretion. Support for this model included experimental evidence of functional CCK receptors on rat acinar cells that stimulate second messenger systems and amylase release. In addition, CCK stimulates pancreatic enzyme secretion after vagotomy or autotransplantation of the pancreas, suggesting that neural mechanisms were less important. This simplistic model has now been questioned because at physiologic concentrations the action of CCK can be completely blocked by either CCK-A receptor antagonists or muscarinic receptor antagonists. Secondly, human pancreatic acinar cells appear to lack the CCK-A receptor in hormone-binding studies, and the CCK-A receptor messenger RNA is also absent, which means that human acinar cells do not have CCK-A receptors. This and other evidence suggest that CCK works through a neural mechanism rather than directly at the level of the pancreatic acinar cells. Ach—acetylcholine; ATP—adenosine triphosphate; cAMP—cyclic adenosine monophosphate.

FIGURE 1-18.

Physiologic levels of cholecystokinin (CCK) evoke pancreatic enzyme secretion predominantly through cholinergic pathways in humans. The exocrine enzyme response of the pancreas to a meal or CCK infusion is blocked by the muscarinic receptor blocker, atropine. In this example, human volunteers received infusions of CCK with or without atropine, as pancreatic trypsin secretion levels were measured. CCK infusions of 10 pmol/kg/hr result in plasma CCK levels seen after a meal whereas higher infusion rates result in supraphysiologic levels. At physiologic levels of CCK, the pancreatic trypsin output is almost completely blocked, indicating that CCK may be acting through neural mechanisms. The use of rat pancreatic acinar cells (which differ from human pancreatic acinar cells because they express the CCK-A receptor) and the use of supraphysiologic doses of CCK has led to some confusion on the physiologic mechanism controlling pancreatinc secretion. (*Adapted from* Soudah *et al.* [7].)

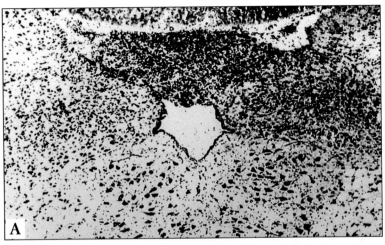
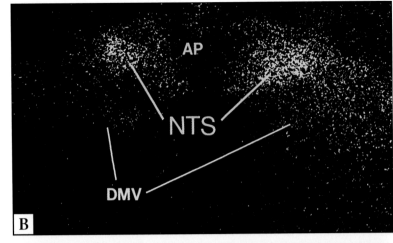
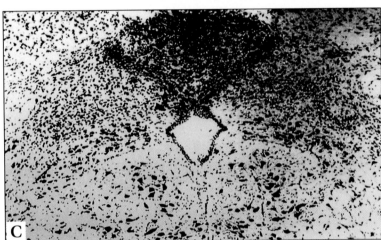
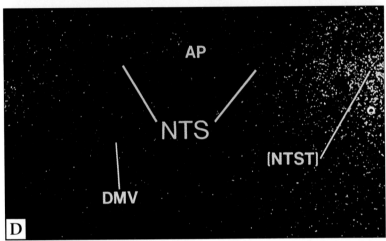

Cholecystokinin (CCK) receptors are on the terminal fields of afferent vagal fibers. Intravenous infusion of CCK results in a number of central nervous system actions that are blocked with disruption of the afferent (sensory) vagal fibers. During the 1980s CCK-A receptors were demonstrated on vagal afferent (sensory) fibers. **A,** A cross-section of a rat brain brainstem projection of vagal sensory fibers with CCK-A receptors and the disappearance of these receptors with chemical destruction of the vagal sensory fiber. **B,** Photographic film that was placed over the section in **panel A** when it was incubated with radiolabeled CCK. The radiolabeled CCK bound to CCK receptors,

which are identified by the white spots. The receptors are in the nucleus tractus solitarius (NTS), which is the sensory nerve receptive area for the vagus (described in more detail later). **C,** Photomicrograph of an equivalent area at the brainstem of a rat given intra-abdominal capsaicin to destroy the sensory vagal fibers. **D,** The CCK receptors on the sensory vagal fibers projecting to the sensory receptive area of the brainstem (*ie,* the NTS) are now absent (compare **panel B** and **panel D**), demonstrating that CCK receptors are on vagal fibers and that they project to the sensory receptive region of the brain.

Physiologic evidence that the cholecystokinin (CCK) receptors mediating pancreatic secretion are on afferent (sensory) vagal fibers. This experiment tested the effect of eliminating the sensory arm of the vagus by applying the sensory neurotoxin, capsaicin, to the vagus or duodenum or by transecting the afferent vagal rootlet. CCK infusion at physiologic doses (≤ 40 pmol/kg/h) caused a dose-dependent increase in pancreatic enzyme secretion in the control animals, but application of capsaicin or vagal afferent rootlet section completely abolished the pancreatic response to CCK. Centrally stimulated pancreatic secretion remained intact, proving that the site of CCK's action at physiologic doses was on the afferent vagal fibers (not shown). (*Adapted from* Li *et al.* [8].)

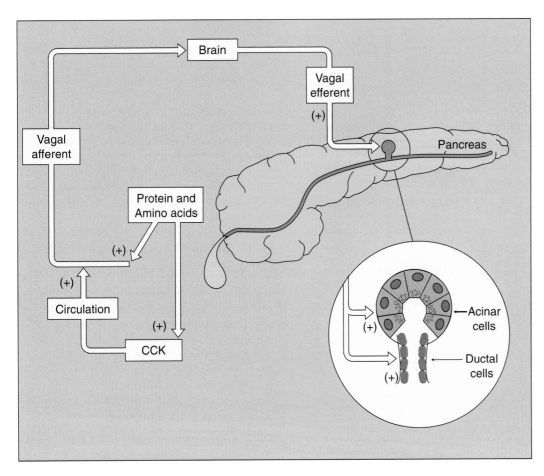

FIGURE 1-21.

The mechanism controlling cholecystokinin (CCK)-stimulated pancreatic secretion must now be modified to include the vagus nerve. A central role of the vagal system in CCK-stimulated pancreatic secretion is supported by current experimental evidence and makes physiologic sense. This modified model illustrates the mechanical advantage of the afferent vagal → efferent vagal → intrapancreatic nerve → acinar cell loop. Thus, a modest release of CCK from the duodenum causes a significant release of digestive enzymes through an amplification of the response in the brainstem and in the intrapancreatic ganglia. Furthermore, this model explains how the response to CCK can be potentiated or inhibited by neuromodulators acting at various sites along the stimulatory pathway.

Release of cholecystokinin-feedback inhibition

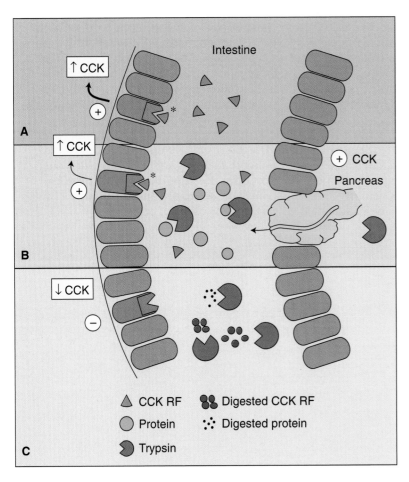

FIGURE 1-22.

A–C, Duodenal release of cholecystokinin (CCK). This diagram helps to explain how proteolytic enzyme secretion from the pancreas completes a negative feedback loop. For over 50 years it has been known that CCK is released into the bloodstream from cells in the duodenal mucosa in the presence of duodenal proteins. Hints as to the mechanism came from the observation that blocking the action of pancreatic enzymes in the duodenum (by diverting the pancreatic juice away from the duodenum or by adding potent protease inhibitors) also caused a potent release of CCK. This, and other evidence, led to speculation that the duodenum contains a peptide called CCK-releasing factor (CCK-RF) that is responsible for stimulating CCK release when protolytic enzyme is abolished by pancreatic juice diversion or with protease inhibitors (**part A**). Two peptides, luminal CCK-RF and diazepam-binding inhibitor, have recently been described that may be the CCK-RF [8a,8b]. Between meals the CCK-RF is quickly hydrolyzed by proteolytic pancreatic enzymes, and therefore does not cause CCK release. When dietary proteins enter the duodenum (**part B**), they competitively inhibit the action of pancreatic enzymes, thus allowing the concentration of CCK-RF to increase and stimulate CCK release. CCK-RF continues to stimulate CCK release, which stimulates pancreatic enzyme secretion, until the ingested proteins and the CCK-RF are hydrolyzed. The CCK-RF stimulus for CCK release is thereby eliminated, CCK levels return to normal, and pancreatic enzyme secretion returns to basal levels.

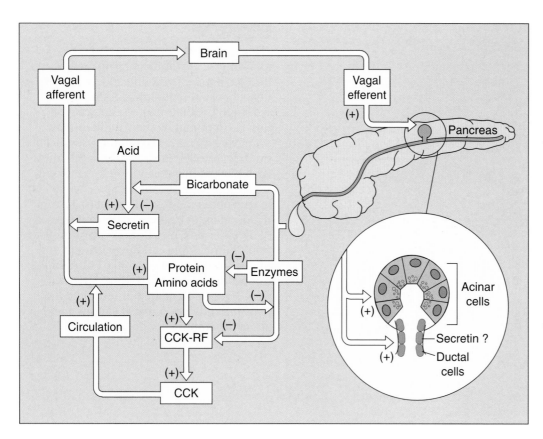

FIGURE 1-23.

Neurohormonal feedback system controlling enzyme secretion. This figure summarizes the major pathways for stimulation and feedback inhibition of pancreatic bicarbonate and enzyme secretion. Duodenal acidification causes release of secretin, which stimulates vagal-vagal and other neural pathways to activate pancreatic duct cells, which in turn secrete bicarbonate-rich fluid. Secretin may also act directly on the ductal cells. The bicarbonate neutralizes the duodenal acid and the feedback loop is completed. Duodenal proteins cause a competitive reduction in free proteolytic enzyme activity, thereby leading to an increase in free cholecystokinin-releasing factor (CCK-RF). The CCK-RF stimulates CCK release into the blood. At physiologic concentrations CCK acts predominantly through vagal-vagal pathways to cause acetylcholine-mediated pancreatic enzyme secretion. The pancreas continues to secrete proteolytic enzymes until the duodenal protein and CCK-RF are digested and the free duodenal proteolytic enzyme activity rises, thus completing another important physiologic feedback loop.

■ PANCREATIC NERVOUS SYSTEM

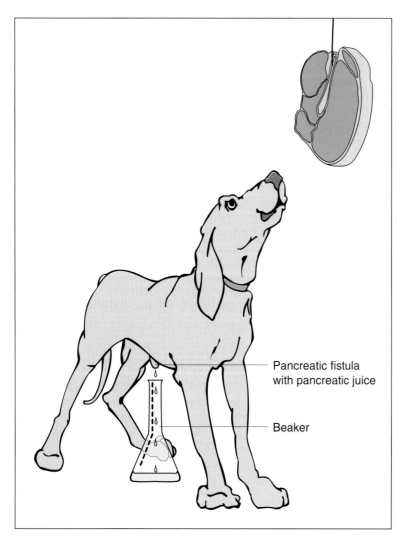

Pancreatic fistula with pancreatic juice

Beaker

FIGURE 1-24.

Most of the fundamental work on nervous innervation of the salivary glands, stomach, and pancreas came from the work of Pavlov and his students. Pavlov's creative surgical techniques allowed him to isolate various aspects of feeding, including "psychological feeding." Thus, the sight or smell of food caused copious flows of gastric juice, which was eliminated by vagotomy and reproduced by stimulation of the peripheral ends of the cut vagi. Perfection of the pancreatic fistula allowed Pavlov to demonstrate that the secretory fibers to the vagus were also within the vagus, but not within the splanchnic nerves. The discovery that duodenal and jejunal acid released secretin rather than acting solely through nervous reflexes diverted attention from the importance of the nervous system in controlling pancreatic secretion. The importance of the nervous system is now being rediscovered, however.

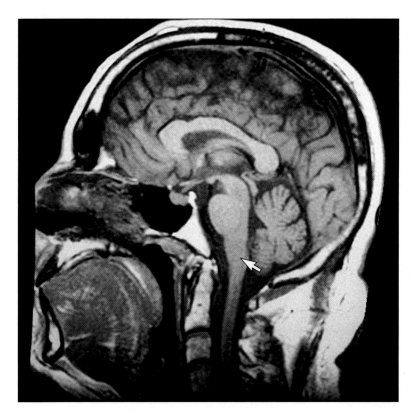

FIGURE 1-25.

MR image of the brain demonstrating the level of the dorsal vagal complex in humans. The central mechanisms culminating in the cephalic phase of pancreatic secretion remain obscure. It is clear, however, that the central response is relayed to the dorsal vagal complex in the brainstem, where central and peripheral inputs are integrated and relayed to the pancreatic ganglia through motor neurons located in the dorsal vagal complex. The dorsal vagal complex (*arrow*) consists of three major components. The dorsal motor nucleus (DMN) of the vagus contains the motor neurons, whose axons project directly to intrapancreatic ganglia. The tractus solitarius is a sensory receptive area. Axons from higher brain centers and sensory vagal fibers from the abdomen terminate within this area. Dendrites from dorsal motor neurons also project to the nucleus of the tractus solitarius (NTS), allowing for monosynaptic vagal-vagal reflexes. The third major component is the area postrema (AP), which is also known as the *chemoreceptor trigger zone*. The AP is one of the few areas of the brain without an intact blood- brain barrier. This feature allows it to function as a sensory area for circulating hormones, neuromodulators, and other bloodborne substances. Heavy crossinnervation exists among the AP, NTS, and DMN.

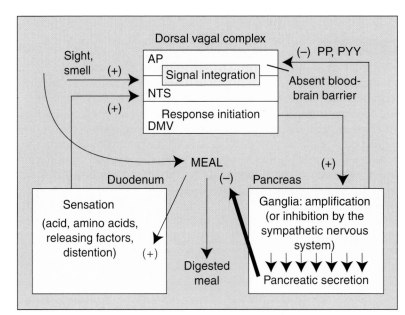

FIGURE 1-26.

Central integration of neurohormonal inputs to the pancreas. Recognition that under physiologic conditions cholecystokinin (CCK) and secretin act predominantly through neural mechanisms has focused attention on the role of the dorsal vagal complex for central integration of stimuli to the pancreas. Central nervous system input from hypothalamic and limbic centers provides strong stimulatory or inhibitory input to the sensory receptive areas. Sensory vagal fibers also project to this area from the gastrointestinal tract. Vagal afferent fibers may be activated directly by luminal distention, amino acids, fatty acids, and sugars, as well as CCK and secretin. The area postrema (the chemoreceptor trigger zone) has an incomplete blood-brain area; therefore, it may provide a mechanism for integrating input from inhibitory hormones and other circulating factors, such as toxins. The integrated sensory input determines the motor output to the pancreas. Further amplification or inhibition also occurs within the pancreas in intrapancreatic ganglia before the stimulatory message finally reaches the ductal and acinar cells.

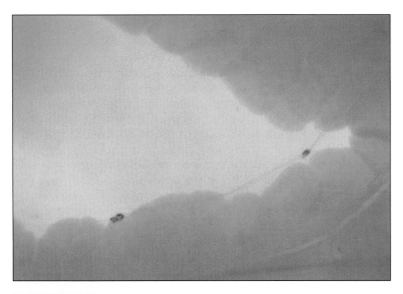

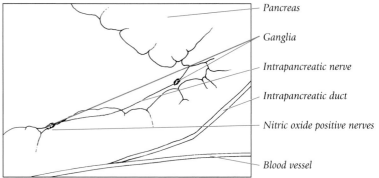

FIGURE 1-27.

Pancreatic ganglia. An extensive network of pancreatic nerves and ganglia spans the pancreatic parenchyma. This figure illustrates two ganglia from a rat pancreas that contain nitric oxide–positive (purple) neurons. Intrapancreatic ganglia receive input from motor nerves arising in dorsal motor nucleus of the vagus, from sympathetic fibers originating in the thoracic spinal cord, and from enteric neurons in the stomach and duodenum. The intrapancre-

atic ganglia serve as the final level of integration, amplification, and modulation. Under physiologic conditions the intrapancreatic ganglia primarily serve a relay function. Under conditions of decentralization (*eg*, vagotomy or transplantation), however, there is some evidence of neuroplasticity, in which these neurons may develop sensitivity to cholecystokinin and other circulating hormones.

TABLE 1-1. INHIBITORY NEUROPEPTIDES

PEPTIDE	MODE OF ACTION	MECHANISM
Glucagon	Endocrine/paracrine	Unknown
Somatostatin	Endocrine/paracrine	Multiple neural
Pancreatic polypeptide	Endocrine/paracrine	(-) Cholinergics
Peptide YY	Endocrine/paracrine	(-) Cholinergics
Neuropeptide Y	Neurocrine	(-) Cholinergics
Enkephalin	Neurocrine	(-) Cholinergics
Calcitonin gene-related peptide	Neurocrine	Unknown
Pancreastatin	Unknown	(-) Cholinergics

TABLE 1-1.

Inhibitory neuromodulators. The neural network controlling pancreatic secretion can be stimulated by higher centers during the cephalic phase of digestion, by sensory fibers in the stomach and duodenum, and through receptors for secretin and cholecystokinin on afferent vagal fibers. In addition, various regulatory peptides inhibit pancreatic secretion. Far less is known about inhibitory peptides than stimulatory hormones; however, it is clear that most act through neural mechanisms. Two of the most important are somatostatin and pancreatic polypeptide.

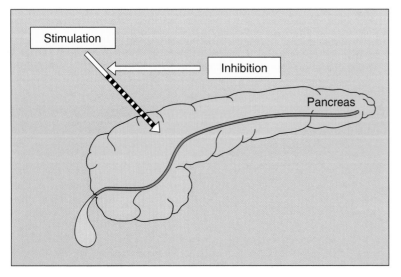

FIGURE 1-28.

The physiologic role of inhibitory peptides and the pathophysiologic consequence of impairing their action have not been fully determined. It appears, however, that the inhibitory neuropeptides actively modulate pancreatic secretion during a meal because immunoneutralization of the inhibitory peptides, somatostatin, pancreatic polypeptide, or peptide YY, results in a 30% to 40% increase in pancreatic output. Two inhibitory peptides that have been widely studied are somatostatin and pancreatic polypeptide.

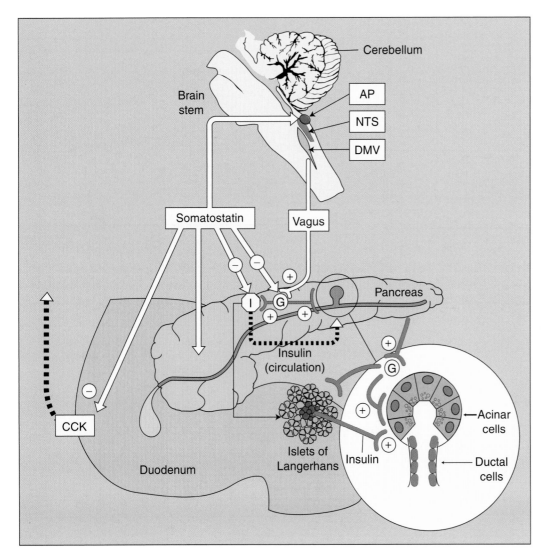

FIGURE 1-29.

Somatostatin inhibits pancreatic secretion at multiple sites. Somatostatin inhibits pancreatic secretion by inhibiting release of stimulatory peptides (*eg*, cholecystokinin) through inhibitory actions at central nervous system sites, by modulating intra-pancreatic ganglia, by inhibiting release of acetylcholine at the presynaptic endplate, and possibly by inhibition of insulin release, which is required for active secretion. Although somatostatin receptors are also found on pancreatic acinar cells, these receptors appear to modulate growth rather than to inhibit enzyme secretion directly. The widespread distribution of somato-statin and its multiple receptor types has made it difficult to determine the exact physiologic role of somatostatin. The powerful effect on inhibiting pancreatic secretion at multiple sites, however, and the clinical availability of somatostatin and long-acting somatostatin congeners (*eg*, octreotide) emphasizes the importance of this system. AP—area postrema; DMV—dorsal motor nucleus of the vagus; NTS—nucleus of the tractus solitarius.

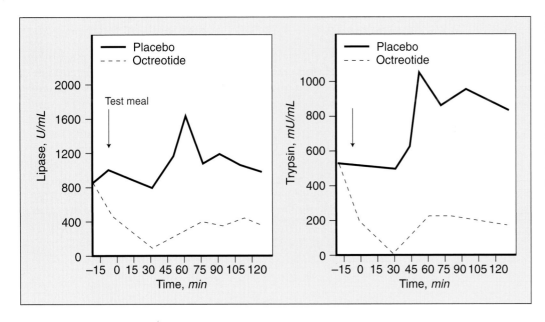

FIGURE 1-30.

The somatostatin receptor agonist, octreotide, inhibits meal-stimulated pancreatic enzyme secretion in humans. These graphs illustrate the effect of octreotide acetate 25 μg or placebo given 15 minutes before a test meal. Lipase and trypsin output were reduced to below basal levels for more than 2 hours after the administration of this clinically available somatostatin receptor agonist. (*Adapted from* Lembcke *et al.* [9].)

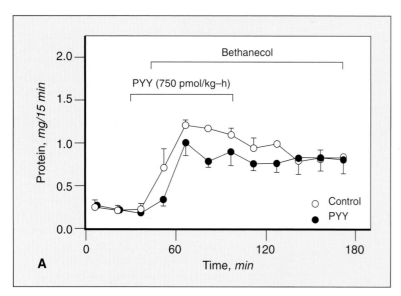

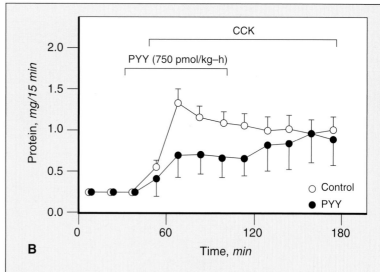

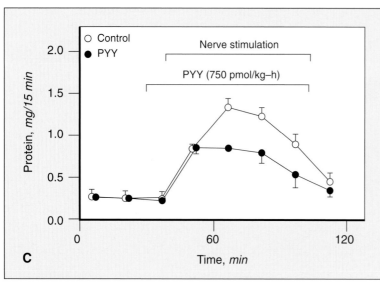

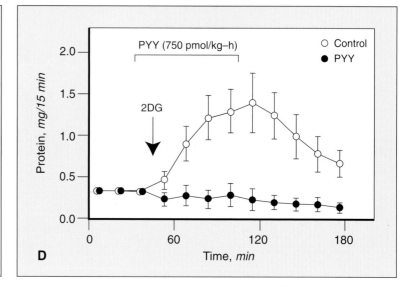

FIGURE 1-31.

Pancreatic polypeptide (PP) and peptide YY (PYY) inhibit pancreatic secretion through indirect mechanisms. These experiments give insight into the mechanism used by PYY (and PP) in the inhibition of pancreatic secretion. Each panel represents a different method of experimentally stimulating the pancreas. **A,** Pancreatic secretion is directly stimulated at the acinar cells with the muscarinic (acetylcholine) receptor agonist, bethanechol. Peptide YY, even at supraphysiologic doses, causes minimal inhibition of pancreatic protein (*ie,* enzyme) secretion. **B,** Pancreatic secretion is stimulated with cholecystokinin (CCK). Because supraphysiologic doses were used, secretion was stimulated by multiple pathways in this experiment (compare to Figure 1-17). Note a partial inhibition of CCK-stimulated pancreatic secretion by large doses of PYY (the partial inhibition

of CCK by PYY may reflect inhibition of vagal-vagal pathways, but not noncholinergic intrapancreatic pathways). **C,** Pancreatic secretion is stimulated through direct electrical stimulation of the distal end of the cut cervical vagus. Again, supraphysiologic doses of PYY cause only a modest inhibition of pancreatic secretion. **D,** Pancreatic secretion stimulated centrally (*ie,* from the hypothalamus) by 2-deoxyglucose (2DG). When pancreatic secretion is stimulated at a site more proximal to the efferent vagus than PYY, at physiologic doses (one tenth of the dose in **panel A, panel B,** or **panel C**) it completely inhibits pancreatic secretion. This and other experiments suggest that PYY and PP modulate stimulatory input to the exocrine pancreas from sites outside the pancreas, proximal to the efferent vagus nerve. (*Adapted from* Putnam *et al.* [10]; with permission.)

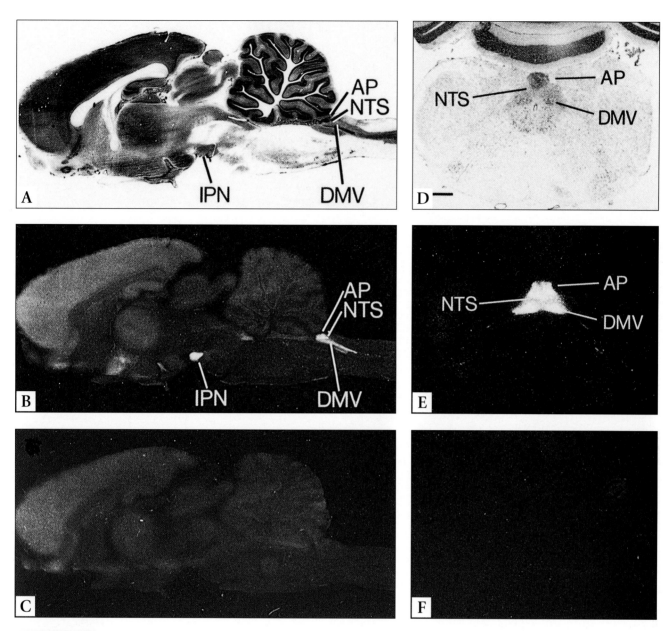

Figure 1-32.

Receptors for pancreatic polypeptides (PP) are located in the dorsal vagal complex. In 1989, receptors for pancreatic polypeptides were discovered in the dorsal vagal complex, including the area postrema (AP), which has an incomplete blood- brain barrier [11]. Localization of PP receptors in the brain of rats is demonstrated in these autoradiographs. The location of the autoradiographs is demonstrated by Nissl stain of midsagittal (**panel A**) and coronal (**panel D**) sections of the rat brain through the dorsal vagal complex. **panel B** and **panel E** are dark-field photomicrographs of the radiosensitive film that overlaid the section in **panel A** and **panel D**. High concentrations of specific ^{125}I-PP binding sites appear white. Binding is observed in the dorsal vagal complex, which includes the AP, nucleus of the tractus solitarius

(NTS), and dorsal motor nucleus of the vagus (DMV). **Panel C** and **panel F** are dark-field photomicrographs of adjacent sections that were incubated with ^{125}I-PP along with unlabeled PP at 1 μmol/L, and thus represent nonspecific binding. Further experiments demonstrated that circulating PP was specifically bound to these sites. This discovery provided an anatomic explanation for the observed remote site of PP's action on the pancreas. The recognition that under physiologic conditions cholecystokinin and secretin act, in large part, through vagal-vagal reflexes passing through the dorsal vagal complex further emphasizes the importance of an inhibitory modulator at this central control site. (**A**, bar=5 mm; **D**, bar=1mm). IPN—interpeduncular nucleus. (*From* Whitcomb [11]; with permission.)

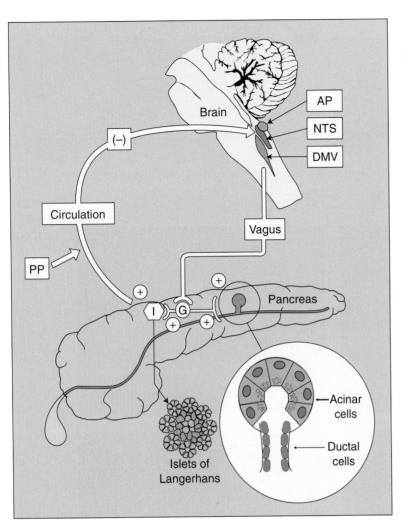

FIGURE 1-33.

Negative feedback for central vagal activity. This figure illustrates the current hypothesis on how pancreatic polypeptides (PP) modulate central vagal activity. First, central or sensory input causes increased vagal motor activity, which initiates pancreatic secretion and also stimulates PP release. As the stimulatory input continues, PP plasma levels rise. PP then circulates to the brainstem, where it crosses the blood-brain barrier at the area postrema (AP) and binds to PP receptors. Activation of the PP receptors inhibits central vagal activity, thus completing a negative feedback loop. DMV—dorsal motor nucleus of the vagus; NTS—nucleus of the tractus solitarious. (*Adapted from* Whitcomb [11]; with permission.)

■ ACKNOWLEDGMENTS

The author would like to thank Melanie B. Fukui, MD for the MR images of the brain, and John Walsh, MD for the CCK antiserum.

■ REFERENCES

1. Bayliss W, Starling E: The mechanism of pancreatic secretion. *J Physiol Lond* 1902, 28:325–353.

2. Malagelada JR, Go VL, Summerskill WH: Different gastric pancreatic, pancreatic, and biliary responses to solid-liquid or homogenized meals. *Dig Dis Sci* 1979, 24:101–110.

2a. Netter FH: Nervous system, part 1. In *The CIBA Collection of Medical Illustrations*, section IV (Anatomy and Physiology). Edited by Brass A. West Caldwell, NJ: CIBA Pharmaceutical Division; 1991:70.

3. Case R, Argent B: Bicarbonate secretion by pancreatic duct cells: Mechanisms and control. In Go W, Gardner J, Brooks F, *et al.* (eds): *The Exocrine Pancreas: Biology, Pathobiology, and Diseases.* New York: Raven Press; 1986:213–243.

4. Harper A, Raper H: Pancreozymin, a stimulant of the secretion of pancreatic enzymes in extracts of the small intestine. *J Physiol Lond* 1943, 102:115–125.

5. Mutt V, Jorpes J: Structure of porcine cholecystokinin-pancreozymin. *Eur J Biochem* 1968, 125:156–162.

6. Ivy A, Oldberg E: A hormone mechanism for gallbladder contraction and evacuation. *Am J Physiol* 1928, 86:599–613.

7. Soudah HC, Lu Y, Hasler WL, Owyang C: Cholecystokinin at physiological levels evokes pancreatic enzyme secretion via a cholinergic pathway. *Am J Physiol* 1992, 263:G102–G107.

8. Li Y, Owyang C: Vagal afferent pathway mediates physiological action of cholecystokinin on pancreatic enzyme secretion. *J Clin Invest* 1993, 92:418–424.

8a. Spannagel A, Green G, Guan D, *et al.*: Purification and characterization of a luminal cholecystokinin-releasing factory from rat intestinal secretion. *Proc Natl Acad Sci USA* 1996, 93:4415–4420.

8b. Herzig K, Schon I, Tatemoto K, *et al.*: Diazepam binding inhibitor is a potent cholecystokinin-releasing peptide in the intestine. *Proc Natl Acad Sci USA* 1996, 93:7927–7932.

9. Lembcke B, Creutzfeldt W, Schleser S, *et al.*: Effect of the somatostatin analogue sandostatin (SMS 201-995) in gastrointestinal, pancreatic and biliary function and hormone release in normal men. *Digestion* 1987, 36:108–124.

10. Putnam WS, Liddle RA, Williams JA: Inhibitory regulation of rat pancreas by peptide YY and pancreatic polypeptide. *Am J Physiol* 1989, 256:G698–G703.

11. Whitcomb DC, Taylor IL: A new twist in the brain-gut axis. *Am J Med Sci* 1992, 304:334–338.

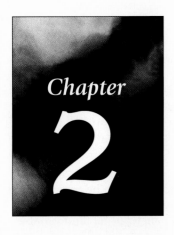

Chapter 2

Pathogenesis of Pancreatic Diseases

JAMES H. GRENDELL

Acute pancreatitis, chronic pancreatitis (with or without pancreatic insufficiency), and pancreatic cancer (adenocarcinoma) are common diseases in industrialized nations. Although etiologies and risk factors for these disorders can often be identified, the pathogenesis of pancreatitis and pancreatic cancer is not well understood. In this chapter, theories of pathogenesis of pancreatic disease are reviewed and illustrated. The reader should also refer to other chapters in the volume for more detailed information on the clinical aspects of pancreatitis and pancreatic cancer.

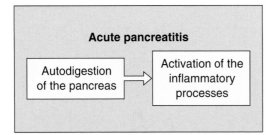

Acute pancreatitis

Autodigestion of the pancreas → Activation of the inflammatory processes

FIGURE 2-1.

Acute pancreatitis was described by Chiari [1] a century ago as an autodigestion of the gland. Chiari proposed that premature activation within the pancreas of its normally secreted digestive enzymes results in inflammation and necrosis of pancreatic tissue. Recently, it has become increasingly clear that it is the secondary involvement of a variety of inflammatory processes, both within and outside the pancreas, that determines the severity of the disease process.

FIGURE 2-2.

The pathophysiology of acute pancreatitis can be considered as involving three stages. The first stage is pancreatic injury with edema, inflammation, necrosis of pancreatic fat, and variable degrees of necrosis of pancreatic secretory cells. The second stage is spread of the inflammatory process to surrounding tissues, with development of retroperitoneal edema, peripancreatic fat necrosis, and an ileus, with "third spacing" of fluid and electrolytes in the gastrointestinal tract resulting in hemoconcentration (increased hematocrit). The third stage involves systemic complications, such as hypotension/shock, multiorgan system failure (*eg*, respiratory, renal), metabolic disturbances, such as hypoalbuminemia and hypocalcemia, and sepsis.

Pathophysiology of acute pancreatitis

Severity
Mild

↓

Severe

Stage 1. Pancreatic injury
Edema, inflammation, fat necrosis, variable necrosis of pancreatic secretory cells

Stage 2. Local (peripancreatic) effects
Retroperitoneal edema, extensive fat necrosis, ileus with "third-spacing" of fluid and electrolytes

Stage 3. Systemic complications
Hypotension/shock, metabolic disturbances, organ failure, sepsis

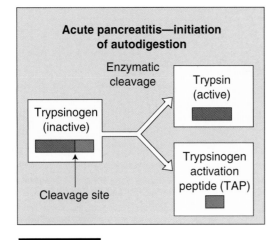

Acute pancreatitis—initiation of autodigestion

Trypsinogen (inactive) → Enzymatic cleavage → Trypsin (active)

→ Trypsinogen activation peptide (TAP)

Cleavage site

FIGURE 2-3.

For autodigestion to occur, it is likely that the key initiating step is the conversion of the zymogen (digestive enzyme precursor), trypsinogen, to its enzymatically active form, trypsin, by cleavage of the small trypsinogen activation peptide (TAP). The mechanism by which this occurs remains uncertain and is the object of intensive investigation; however, activation of trypsinogen to trypsin can be demonstrated at a very early step in the development of acute pancreatitis in experimental animal models. Furthermore, both trypsin and TAP have been demonstrated in the circulation of patients with acute pancreatitis.

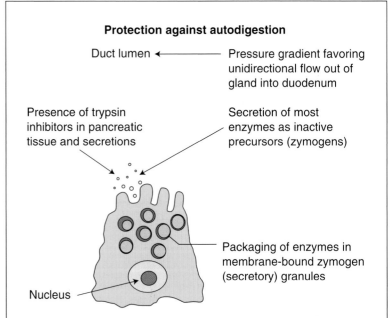

Protection against autodigestion

Duct lumen ← Pressure gradient favoring unidirectional flow out of gland into duodenum

Presence of trypsin inhibitors in pancreatic tissue and secretions

Secretion of most enzymes as inactive precursors (zymogens)

Packaging of enzymes in membrane-bound zymogen (secretory) granules

Nucleus

FIGURE 2-4.

Various protective mechanisms reduce the likelihood of premature activation of trypsinogen to trypsin within the pancreatic parenchyma and initiation of autodigestion of the pancreas. These include the secretion of most digestive enzymes in their inactive precursor forms (as zymogens [*eg*, trypsinogen]) in addition to the packaging of secretory proteins in membrane-bound storage compartments (zymogen granules). Additionally, trypsin inhibitors present in pancreatic tissue, and in pancreatic secretions, can inactivate small amounts of trypsin, if present. Furthermore, the pressure gradient between the pancreatic duct and the bile duct or duodenum favors the flow of pancreatic secretions out of the gland into the duodenum, which mitigates against reflux of bile or duodenal juice into the pancreas.

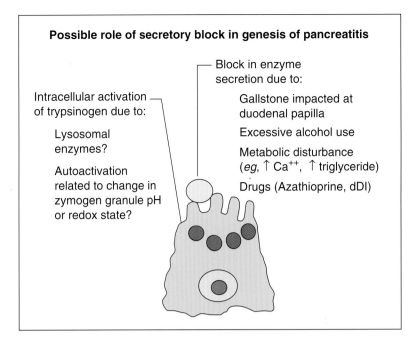

Possible role of secretory block in genesis of pancreatitis

Intracellular activation of trypsinogen due to:

Lysosomal enzymes?

Autoactivation related to change in zymogen granule pH or redox state?

Block in enzyme secretion due to:

Gallstone impacted at duodenal papilla

Excessive alcohol use

Metabolic disturbance (eg, ↑ Ca^{++}, ↑ triglyceride)

Drugs (Azathioprine, dDI)

FIGURE 2-5.

In the clinical setting it is not clear how etiologic factors as diverse as gallstone disease, excessive alcohol use, medications, and metabolic disturbances (*eg,* hypertriglyceridemia, hypercalcemia) can all lead to the development of acute pancreatitis; however, experimental studies in animals and limited data in humans suggest that blockage of digestive enzyme secretion out of the pancreatic acinar cell may be a common predisposing factor. Activation of trypsinogen to trypsin may occur through exposure of trypsinogen to lysosomal enzymes, such as cathepsin B, or alternatively may result from an autoactivation process, perhaps involving an alteration in zymogen granule stability resulting from a change in the pH of the granule or its redox state.

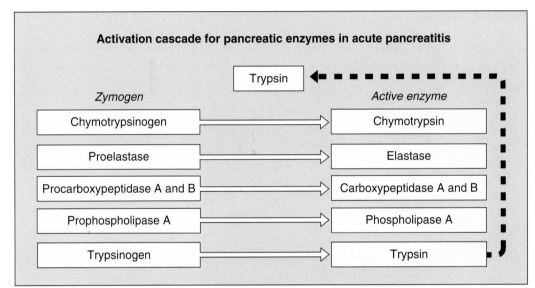

Activation cascade for pancreatic enzymes in acute pancreatitis

Trypsin

Zymogen → *Active enzyme*

Chymotrypsinogen → Chymotrypsin

Proelastase → Elastase

Procarboxypeptidase A and B → Carboxypeptidase A and B

Prophospholipase A → Phospholipase A

Trypsinogen → Trypsin

FIGURE 2-6.

Once trypsin is present in an amount that exceeds the ability of trypsin inhibitor to inactivate it, trypsin can catalyze the activation of other zymogens (*eg,* chymotrypsinogen, proelastase, procarboxypeptidase A and B, prophospholipase A), as well as of trypsinogen itself, initiating the "autodigestion" of the pancreas.

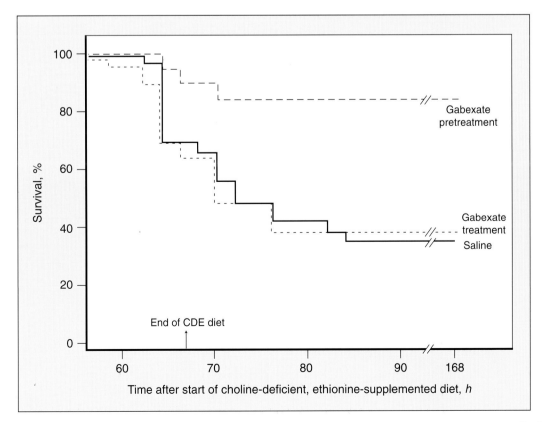

FIGURE 2-7.

Although zymogen activation may be central to the initiation of acute pancreatitis, it does not appear to determine either the extent of pancreatic injury or the severity of the systemic effects. In an experimental model of severe diet-induced acute pancreatitis in mice, pretreatment of animals with the potent trypsin inhibitor, gabexate, markedly reduced mortality whereas treatment of mice with gabexate *after* initiation of pancreatitis had no effect on mortality. Similarly, clinical studies have failed to show a benefit from use of trypsin inhibitors in the treatment of patients with established acute pancreatitis. (*Adapted from* Niederau *et al.* [2]; with permission.)

Pathogenesis of Pancreatic Diseases **2.3**

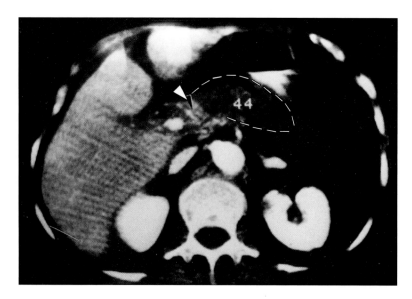

FIGURE 2-8.

Bolus contrast-enhanced computed tomography (CT) in severe acute pancreatitis. A major unsettled issue in the pathophysiology of acute pancreatitis is why most cases are mild and self-limited whereas some progress to the more severe, potentially lethal end of the spectrum of disease. Impairment of the pancreatic microcirculation leading to tissue ischemia may be an important factor in determining the extent of injury and necrosis of the pancreas and the ultimate severity of the disease process. A clinical correlate of this tissue ischemia may be failure of the pancreas to enhance in density on CT after intravenous injection of a bolus of a CT contrast agent in patients with more severe acute pancreatitis. (*Arrowhead*—Normally enhancing tissue in neck of pancreas; *outlined area*—Nonenhancing body and tail of the pancreas.)

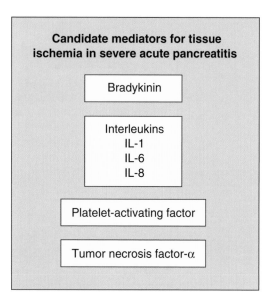

Candidate mediators for tissue ischemia in severe acute pancreatitis

Bradykinin

Interleukins IL-1 IL-6 IL-8

Platelet-activating factor

Tumor necrosis factor-α

FIGURE 2-9.

Factors which may be important in deranging the microcirculation in the pancreas include bradykinin, oxygen-derived free radicals, interleukins (IL) (*eg*, IL-1, IL-6, IL-8), platelet-activating factor, and tumor necrosis factor-α.

Cellular sources of inflammatory mediators in acute pancreatitis

Early

Tissue macrophages in the pancreas: IL-1, IL-6, IL-8, TNF-α

Endothelial cells: IL-8, PAF

T-helper lymphocytes: IL-2, interferon-γ

Late

TABLE 2-1. POTENTIAL FACTORS CONTRIBUTING TO THE SYSTEMIC MANIFESTATIONS OF ACUTE PANCREATITIS

Oxygen-derived free radicals

Bradykinin

Pro-inflammatory cytokines (IL-1, IL-6, IL-8, tumor necrosis factor-α, platelet-activating factor)

Complement

TABLE 2-1.

Some of the systemic effects in severe pancreatitis (*eg*, multiorgan system failure, acute respiratory distress syndrome, "capillary leak" syndrome) resemble those observed in patients with sepsis, severe traumatic injury, and extensive burns (systemic inflammatory response syndrome [SIRS]). A variety of inflammatory mediators and cytokines activated following the initial injury to the pancreas appear to be involved in this process, "amplifying" the effects of pancreatic autodigestion throughout the body. Potentially important factors include oxygen-derived free radicals, bradykinin and other vasoactive substances, cytokines, acute phase reactants (proinflammatory cytokines), and components of the complement system. IL—interleukin.

FIGURE 2-10.

In the early stages of pancreatic injury and inflammation, proinflammatory cytokines, such as interleukin (IL)-1, IL-6, IL-8, and tumor necrosis factor (TNF)-α, appear to be released from tissue macrophages within the pancreas. Neutrophil activation likely results from release of IL-8 from macrophages and endothelial cells and release of platelet-activating factor (PAF) from endothelial cells. Later in the process, release of cytokines from T-helper lymphocytes (*eg*, IL-2, interferon-γ) may also participate in the inflammatory response [3].

TABLE 2-2. POTENTIAL DEFENSE MECHANISMS IN ACUTE PANCREATITIS

Antioxidants (gluthione and other compounds containing sulfhydryl groups)
Anti-inflammatory cytokines (eg, IL-2, IL-10, IL-1 receptor antagonist)
Others?

TABLE 2-2.

Because clinical acute pancreatitis is usually a relatively mild and self-limited disease, defense mechanisms must exist for protecting the pancreas from severe injury and for terminating the inflammatory process; however, these defense mechanisms are currently poorly understood. Antioxidants, such as glutathione and other sulfhydryl-containing compounds in the pancreas, appear to be able to protect the pancreas from injury from oxygen-derived free radicals. Anti-inflammatory cytokines, such as interleukin (IL)-2, IL-10, and IL-1 receptor antagonist may be important in modulating the inflammatory response in a beneficial way. It is likely that other defense mechanisms limiting pancreatic injury will be discovered in the near future.

CHRONIC PANCREATITIS

TABLE 2-3. ANATOMIC-PATHOLOGIC HALLMARKS OF CHRONIC PANCREATITIS

Inflammation
Atrophy of secretory tissue
Fibrosis
Strictures of pancreatic duct (not in all cases)
Duct calculi (not in all cases)

TABLE 2-3.

Any theory concerning the pathophysiology of chronic pancreatitis must account for its well-established morphologic features: chronic inflammation, atrophy of secretory tissue, fibrosis, and in some cases, strictures of the pancreatic duct and duct calculi.

TABLE 2-4. PATHOPHYSIOLOGY OF CHRONIC ALCOHOLIC PANCREATITIS

Must in some way relate to effects of long-term excessive alcohol use on one or more of the following:
    Metabolism of pancreatic secretory cells
    Composition of pancreatic juice
    Secretory pressure in the pancreatic duct
    Sphincter of Oddi function

TABLE 2-4.

Because alcohol use is the primary etiology of chronic pancreatitis in industrialized countries, proposed pathophysiologic mechanisms must relate to effects of chronic excessive use on the pancreas. Alcohol may damage the pancreas by interfering with the metabolism of pancreatic secretory cells, by altering the composition of pancreatic juice, or by affecting the secretory pressure in the pancreatic duct or the function of the sphincter of Oddi.

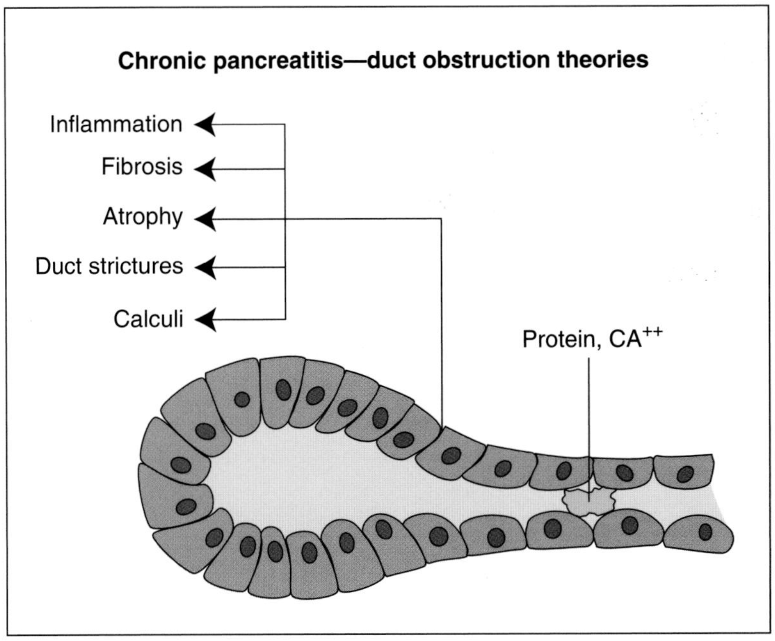

FIGURE 2-11.

One theory [4] proposes that heavy alcohol use leads to a change in the composition of pancreatic juice, resulting in precipitation of plugs (initially in the smaller pancreatic ducts) containing proteins and calcium salts. These plugs may obstruct the ducts, causing inflammation, fibrosis, and atrophy of the secretory tissue. According to this theory, chronic pancreatitis is initially a "duct-based" disease, and may ultimately lead to ductal strictures and calculi within the ductal system.

Chronic pancreatitis—duct obstruction theories

Inflammation
Fibrosis
Atrophy
Duct strictures
Calculi

Protein, CA^{++}

TABLE 2-5. CHRONIC PANCREATITIS: PROTEIN COMPONENTS OF PANCREATIC DUCTAL CALCULI

Lithostathine (pancreatic stone protein)

    Proposed inhibitor of calcium salt precipitation in pancreatic juice; deficiency may → plug formation → chronic pancreatitis

GP-2

    Most abundant protein in zymogen granule membrane, commonly found in ductal plugs

TABLE 2-5.

According to some proponents of the theory given in Figure 2-11, a reduction in the secretion into pancreatic juice of a protein called *lithostathine* is, at least in part, responsible for precipitation of ductal plugs in chronic alcohol-induced pancreatitis, and perhaps other etiologies of pancreatitis as well. Lithostathine has been proposed to act as an inhibitor of calcium salt precipitation in pancreatic juice. Another secreted protein, the glycoprotein GP-2, has also been suggested as a possible factor in intraductal plug formation; however, there is as yet no conclusive evidence for a primary role for either molecule in the pathogenesis of chronic pancreatitis.

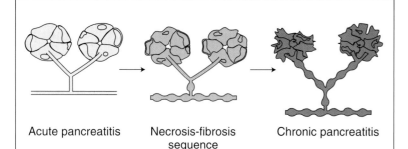

Acute pancreatitis   Necrosis-fibrosis sequence   Chronic pancreatitis

FIGURE 2-12.

An alternative concept [5] is that chronic pancreatitis results from either repetitive acute injury to the pancreas or, perhaps, continuous subclinical injury produced by factors such as alcohol consumption. Cell necrosis and resulting inflammation over time lead to fibrosis and atrophy of pancreatic tissue and to secondary damage to pancreatic ducts. This has been called the *necrosis-fibrosis sequence*, and is analogous to proposed theories describing the development of cirrhosis of the liver as a consequence of chronic hepatitis due to a variety of causes, including viruses and alcohol. This theory is also lacking definitive proof.

TABLE 2-6. PATHOPHYSIOLOGY OF CHRONIC PANCREATITIS

Duct obstruction vs. necrosis-fibrosis

    Different mechanisms in different patients?

    Different mechanisms at different stages of disease in the same patient?

TABLE 2-6.

It is not clear which of these proposed pathophysiologic theories (duct obstruction versus necrosis-fibrosis) most closely explains the development of clinical chronic pancreatitis. It is possible that both may be involved, with one or the other predominating in different patients or at different stages of the disease in the same patient.

CANCER OF THE PANCREAS

TABLE 2-7. CANCER OF THE PANCREAS: PATHOLOGY

90% are adenocarcinomas that appear to arise from duct epithelium

It is believed that cancers are preceded by hyperplastic and dysplastic changes related to chronic inflammation (*eg*, chronic pancreatitis) and effects of carcinogens (*eg*, tobacco smoke)

TABLE 2-7.

About 90% of pancreatic cancers are adenocarcinomas that appear to arise from epithelium of the pancreatic ducts. It has been proposed that the transition from normal cell growth to overt cancer is preceded by hyperplastic and dysplastic changes that are likely related to the presence of chronic inflammation (*eg*, chronic pancreatitis), the effects of carcinogens (*eg*, components of tobacco smoke), or both.

TABLE 2-8. CANCER OF THE PANCREAS: RECEPTORS

Pancreatic tissue contains many receptors for hormones or growth factors
Advanced tumor stage and decreased survival rates have been linked to
  Presence of aFGF, bFGF
  Increase in receptors for TGF-β_2

TABLE 2-8.

Various receptors for a variety of hormones or growth factors have been identified in pancreatic tissue. Some of these may play important roles in pancreatic tumorgenesis. For example, in clinical pancreatic cancer, the presence of either acidic or basic fibroblast growth factor (aFGF, bFGf) or an increase in receptors for transforming growth factor (TGF)–β_2 has been found to be correlated with advanced tumor stage and decreased patient survival rates [6].

TABLE 2-9. CANCER OF THE PANCREAS: GENETIC ALTERATIONS

Codon 12 mutation, K-*ras* oncogene (85%–90%)
p 53 tumor-suppressor gene
DCC gene
APC gene
CD44 gene (may be related to metastatic potential)

TABLE 2-9.

As with other tumors, a number of different genetic alterations have been observed in pancreatic cancer. The most common is a single point mutation at codon 12 of the K-*ras* oncogene, present in 85% to 90% of pancreatic cancers. Analysis for this mutation in aspiration pancreatic biopsy specimens, pancreatic or duodenal juice, or possibly, peripheral blood, may ultimately provide a sensitive and specific means of diagnosing early pancreatic cancers. Although less common than K-*ras* mutations, mutation in the p53 tumor supressor gene, the deleted colon cancer (DCC) gene, the adenomatous polyposis (APC) gene, and the gene expressing the glycoprotein CD44 (a putative adhesion molecule), have all been described in cancers of the pancreas, and may play roles in local disease progression, and in the case of CD44, the tendency to metastasize [6].

TABLE 2-10. CANCER OF THE PANCREAS: POTENTIAL DEVELOPMENTS IN CELL AND MOLECULAR BIOLOGY

Improved early diagnosis?
Inhibitors of cell growth?
Gene therapy?

TABLE 2-10.

Improvements in the understanding of the cell biology of factors regulating growth and differentiation in the pancreas and in the molecular biology of tumorgenesis have the potential to lead to important advances in diagnosis and to possible exciting break-throughs in gene therapy and therapy involving strategies directed at inhibiting cell growth.

REFERENCES

1. Chiari H: Uber die selbstverdauung des manslichen pankreas. *Z Heik* 1986, 17:69–77.
2. Niederau C, Liddle RA, Ferrell LD, Grendell JH: Beneficial effects of CCK-receptor blockade and inhibition of proteolytic enzyme activity in experimental acute hemorrhagic pancreatitis in mice: Evidence for cholecystokinin as a major factor in the development of acute pancreatitis. *J Clin Invest* 1986, 78:1056–1063.
3. Kusske AM, Rungione AJ, Reber HA: Cytokines and acute pancreatitis. *Gastroenterology* 1996, 110:649–642.
4. Sarles H, Bernhard JP, Johnson CD: Pathogenesis and epidemiology of chronic pancreatitis. *Ann Rev Med* 1989, 40:453–468.
5. Ammann RW, Heitz PU, Kloppel G: Course of alcoholic chronic pancreatitis: A prospective clinicomorphological long-term study. *Gastroenterology* 1996, 111:224–231.
6. Freedman SD, Waxman I: Biology of pancreatic cancer. In *Gastrointestinal Cancers: Biology, Diagnosis, and Therapy.* Edited by Rustgi AK. Philadelphia: Lippincott-Raven; 1995:315–323.

Chapter

3

Acute Pancreatitis

William M. Steinberg

Acute pancreatitis is a common disorder whose pathogenesis remains obscure. On a worldwide basis, gallstones are the leading etiologic cause, followed by alcoholism. Idiopathic pancreatitis and miscellaneous causes (metabolic, drugs, hereditary pancreatitis, trauma, etc.) account for the remainder.

The diagnosis of acute pancreatitis is usually made using serologic tests, with the lipase assay being more sensitive and specific than the amylase. Elevations of the liver enzyme profile (especially the alanine aminotransferase) on admission point to gallstones as the etiology. Sonography is the best imaging technique for diagnosing gallstone pancreatitis, although during the acute attack its sensitivity is only 70% to 80%. Computed tomography (CT) is reserved for later use to determine if pancreatic necrosis is present, if there is any question of the diagnosis, to look for tumors as an unusual cause of pancreatitis, or to monitor for fluid collections during the second week of hospitalization.

The Ranson and APACHE criteria are commonly used in this country to monitor for severity of pancreatitis. In the United Kingdom and Europe, the modified Glasgow criteria or the serum C reactive protein concentration are used for this purpose.

Acute pancreatitis tends to be a mild disease most often, but complications can occur in up to 25% of patients, with a mortality of 8% to 9%. Early complications during the first week include cardiopulmonary or renal failure and metabolic alterations, such as hypocalcemia, hyperglycemia, and acidosis. Later complications include pancreatic infection from infected necrosis and other more uncommon entities.

Principles of management include giving nothing by mouth, continual analgesia, large amounts of intravenous fluid and electrolytes, and treatment of any complications. In the past few years, certain specific therapies have also proven promising. Emergency endoscopic retrograde cholangiopancreatography (ERCP) in suspected gallstone pancreatitis, with removal of stones from the common duct, may improve the prognosis of severe pancreatitis, and does not seem to worsen mild pancreatitis. The antimicrobial drug, imipenem, given soon after admission reduces pancreatic and nonpancreatic infection in severe necrotizing pancreatitis. Peritoneal dialysis for 2 to 3 days continues to be used in some centers to ameliorate multiorgan failure despite two controlled studies showing no efficacy. A recent study employing dialysis for 7 days showed a reduction in the incidence of pancreatic abscess. These results need to be confirmed. The role of surgical débridement in severe pancreatitis needs to be refined. Two retrospective reviews showed no survival benefit for debridement in patients with sterile necrosis. Infected necrosis documented by fine-needle aspiration of the pancreas is a bona fide surgical indication, although the natural history of infected necrosis treated medically is unknown.

ETIOLOGY

TABLE 3-1. ETIOLOGIES

Obstructive
Toxins/drugs
Metabolic
Infection
Vascular
Trauma
Idiopathic

TABLE 3-1.

Etiologic classification of acute pancreatitis. Causes can be divided into obstructive, drug/toxin/metabolic, hereditary, infectious, vascular, traumatic, and idiopathic causes.

TABLE 3-2. OBSTRUCTIVE CAUSES

Gallstones
Ampullary/pancreatic cancer
Worms in pancreatic duct—ascaris
Choledochocele
Periampullary duodenal diverticula
Foreign body obstructing duct
Pancreas divisum with obstruction of accessory papilla
Hypertensive sphincter of Oddi

TABLE 3-2.

Obstructive causes of acute pancreatitis. These include gallstones, ampullary or pancreatic cancer, worms, such as *Ascaris*, choledochocele, periampullary duodenal diverticula, foreign body obstructing the pancreatic duct, pancreas divisum with obstruction of the minor papilla, and hypertensive sphincter of Oddi. By far, the most common cause is gallstones.

TABLE 3-3. TOXINS

Ethyl alcohol
Methyl alcohol
Scorpion toxin
Organophosphorus insecticides

TABLE 3-3.

Toxins causing acute pancreatitis. These include ethyl alcohol, methyl alcohol, scorpion toxin, and organophosphorous insecticides. By far, the most common cause is ethyl alcohol (ethanol).

TABLE 3-4. MAJOR DRUGS THAT CAUSE PANCREATITIS

WITH RECHALLENGES	WITH CONSISTENT LATENCIES
Alpha methyl dopa	Acetaminophen
5-Aminosalicylate	(dDI)
Azathioprine/6 mercaptopurine	Estrogens
Cimetidine	
Furosemide	
Metronidazole	
Pentamidine	
Sulfa drugs	
Sulindac	
Tetracycline	
Valproic acid	
Erythromycin	

TABLE 3-4.

Drugs that can cause acute pancreatitis. These can be divided into two groups. The first group includes those in whom a positive rechallenge with the drug has led to recurrent pancreatitis. Examples of these include azathioprine, pentamidine, and valproic acid.

The second group does not have a positive rechallenge reported, but does have a consistent latency (period of time between exposure of the drug and episode of pancreatitis). Examples in this second group are dideoxyinosine (dDI), acetaminophen, and estrogens. Estrogens may cause pancreatitis by inducing hypertriglyceridemia.

TABLE 3-5. METABOLIC CAUSES

Hypercalcemia—rare

Hypertrigliceridemia—type I, type IV, type V

TABLE 3-5.

Metabolic causes of acute pancreatitis. These are due to hypercalcemia (from whatever cause) and familial or acquired hypertriglyceridemia (triglyceride levels > 1000 mg/dL).

TABLE 3-6. INHERITED (HEREDITARY) PANCREATITIS

Autosomal dominant—abnormal gene or chromosome 7g

Associated with chronic pancreatitis and cancer of the pancreas

TABLE 3-6.

Inherited forms of acute pancreatitis, or *hereditary pancreatitis*. Also referred to as *familial pancreatitis*, these are rare and are passed on by autosomal dominant transmission. These subjects frequently develop chronic pancreatitis over time, and have an increased risk of developing cancer of the pancreas. (*see* chapter on Hereditary Pancreatitis in this volume.)

TABLE 3-7. INFECTIOUS CAUSES OF ACUTE PANCREATITIS

Viruses

    Mumps, cytomegalovirus

    Herpes, hepatitis A, B, C

Bacteria

    Mycobacteria (tuberculosis, *Mycobacterium-avium* complex)

    Leptospirosis

Fungi

    Cryptococcus, Candida, coccidioidomycosis

Parasites

    Ascaris, Clonorchis, Pneumocystis

TABLE 3-7.

Infectious causes of pancreatitis. These are rare, and can be divided into those caused by viruses (*eg*, mumps, cytomegalovirus, etc.); bacteria (tuberculosis, *Mycobacteria-avium* complex, and leptospirosis); fungi, such as *Cryptococcus*, which can cause microabscesses in the pancreas; and parasites, such as *Ascaris*, which are a common source of pancreatitis in underdeveloped countries, where these parasites are highly prevalent.

TABLE 3-8. VASCULAR/HYPOTENSION

Atherosclerotic emboli

Ischemia—hypoperfusion

Vasculitis—systemic lupus erythematosus, polyarteritis

TABLE 3-8.

Vascular causes of pancreatitis. These are due to atherosclerotic emboli to the pancreatic arterial tree, episodes of severe hypotension, or vasculitis (*eg*, in systemic lupus erythematosus).

TABLE 3-9. TRAUMATIC CAUSES OF ACUTE PANCREATITIS

Blunt trauma

Penetrating trauma

Postoperative

Endoscopic retrograde cholangiopancreatography

Sphincter of Oddi manometry

TABLE 3-9.

Traumatic causes of acute pancreatitis. These include blunt trauma to the pancreas (*eg*, steering wheel injury during an automobile accident), and penetrating trauma, as well as iatrogenic trauma to the pancreas (surgical, endoscopic retrograde cholangiopancreatography [ERCP]–induced, or sphincter of Oddi manometry–induced). ERCP-induced pancreatitis occurs in 1% to 10% of these procedures, and performance of sphincter of Oddi manometry doubles or triples this risk.

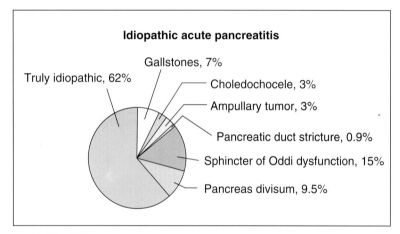

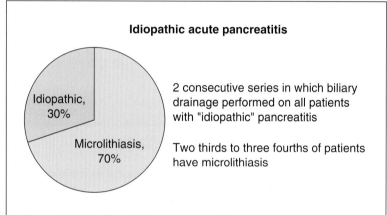

FIGURE 3-1.

"Idiopathic" acute pancreatitis. Final etiologies of cases of idiopathic pancreatitis referred to the Medical College of Wisconsin. After endoscopic retrograde cholangiopancreatography and sphincter of Oddi manometry were performed, 38% of cases were no longer classified as idiopathic, but 62% remained in this category. (*Data from* Venu *et al.* [1].)

FIGURE 3-2.

Biliary drainage of idiopathic acute pancreatitis. In two series of consecutive patients with idiopathic pancreatitis—one from Seattle, the other from Spain—in which biliary drainage was performed, the majority of patients had microlithiasis as the probable cause of pancreatitis. These patients responded to ursodeoxycholic acid (Ursodiol), endoscopic sphincterotomy, or cholecystectomy, with a reduction in the frequency of attacks of pain [2,3].

TABLE 3-10. IDIOPATHIC ACUTE RECURRENT PANCREATITIS

TABLE 3-10.

Use of endoscopic retrograde cholangiopancreatography (ERCP) with sphincter of Oddi (SO) manometry can reduce the number of idiopathic cases, as demonstrated in these two series [1].

ERCP, SO MANOMETRY FINDINGS	VENU (*N*=116)	SHERMAN (*N*=55)	TOTAL (*N*=171)
SO dysfunction	15%	33%	20%
Pancreas divisum	10%	15%	11%
Duct stones	7%	6%	6%
Choledochocele	3%	4%	4%
Tumor (malignant/benign)	3%	5%	4%
Total abnormal	38%	63%	45%

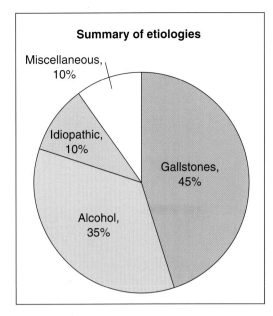

Summary of etiologies

Miscellaneous, 10%

Idiopathic, 10%

Alcohol, 35%

Gallstones, 45%

FIGURE 3-3.

Summary of the main etiologies for acute pancreatitis. A compilation of many studies from around the world reveals that gallstones account for 45% of cases, alcoholism for 35% of cases, miscellaneous causes for 10% of cases, and idiopathic for 10% of cases.

PATHOGENESIS

TABLE 3-11. PATHOGENESIS OF ACUTE PANCREATITIS: INITIATING EVENT UNKNOWN

? Intra-acinar activation of trypsin, which in turn activates chymotrypsin, elastase, and phospholipase A_2

? Accumulation of lipase in interstitium, which leads to peripancreatic fat necrosis

TABLE 3-11.

Pathogenetic sequence of acute pancreatitis. It is presumed that some initiating event causes intra-acinar activation of trypsin, which in turn activates other enzymes leading to cell destruction. Release of lipase into the peripancreatic interstitium leads to peripancreatic fat necrosis.

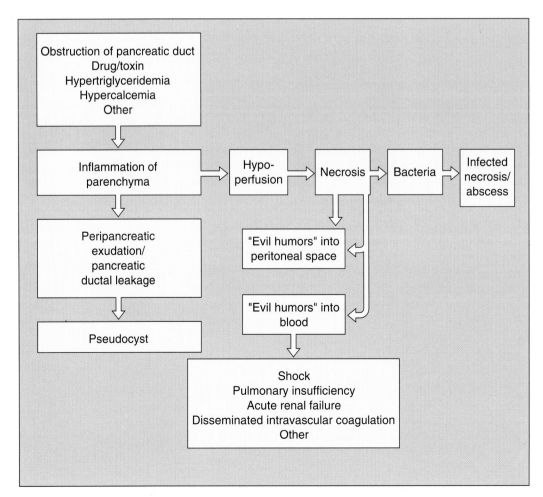

FIGURE 3-4.

Possible pathogenetic sequence of acute pancreatitis. After the acinar cell is triggered, it provokes an intense inflammatory response in the pancreas. Weeping of pancreatic juice into the peripancreatic space or microperforations of the pancreatic ductal system can lead to pseudocyst formation. Subsequent hypoperfusion to the gland can convert mild edematous/interstitial pancreatitis to necrotizing pancreatitis. At this point, release of toxic factors into the systemic circulation, such as trypsin, elastase, phospholipase A_2, and platelet-activating factor or other cytokines, can lead to cardiovascular and pulmonary collapse. The necrotic pancreas can become secondarily infected from hematogenous or transperitoneal sources [4].

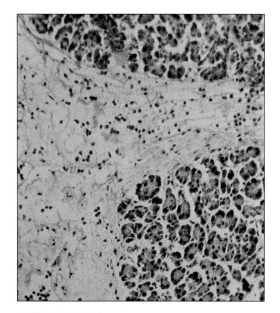

FIGURE 3-5.

Pathology of acute interstitial pancreatitis. There are two main types of acute pancreatitis: interstitial and necrotizing. Interstitial (or edematous) pancreatitis is shown in this photomicrograph. Interstitial pancreatitis is usually associated with clinically mild disease [5].

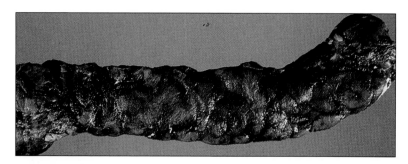

FIGURE 3-6.

Pathology of necrotizing pancreatitis. Extensive ischemic-hemorrhagic necrosis is present in this gross pathology specimen (*From* Klatt [6]; with permission.)

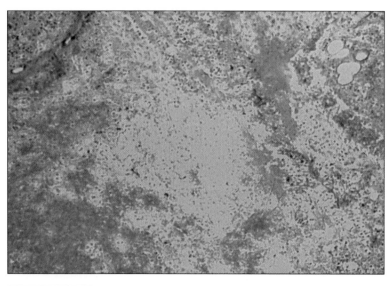

FIGURE 3-7.

Pathology of necrotizing/hemorrhagic pancreatitis. Extensive hemorrhagic necrosis is present. This type of pancreatitis is associated with anemia due to pancreatic hemorrhage and a high mortality rate. Elastase may play a role in hemorrhage. (*From* American Gastroenterological Association [AGA] Collection; with permission.)

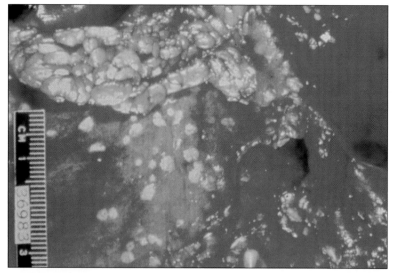

FIGURE 3-8.

Fat necrosis. Fat necrosis seen at surgery is associated with peripancreatic release of lipase, with hydrolysis of triacylglycerols (triglycerides) to toxic fatty acids. (*From* American Gastroenterological Association [AGA] Collection; with permission.)

DIAGNOSIS

TABLE 3-12. DIAGNOSIS OF ACUTE PANCREATITIS

Serum lipase

Serum amylase

Urinary trypsinogen-2

Serum alanine aminotransferase/aspartate aminotransferase

Sonography of gallbladder, common duct

Dynamic (bolus) computed tomographic scan

TABLE 3-12.

Diagnosis of acute pancreatitis. Serum lipase, when threefold or more elevated, is more sensitive and specific than serum amylase in diagnosing pancreatitis. Mild (one- to twofold) elevations of lipase, however, are nonspecific. Threefold increases in alanine aminotransferase or aspartate aminotransferase are highly predictive of gallstone pancreatitis. Sonography should be commonly employed to determine the presence of gallstones, but sonography only has a 70% sensitivity in acute pancreatitis (poorer sensitivity than is seen with gallstones in the absence of acute pancreatitis). Dynamic computed tomography is useful on day 4 or 5 of hospitalization or thereafter in a patient who is seriously ill to look for complications such as necrosis, a developing pseudocyst, or as a prelude to fine-needle aspiration of the pancreas when infection is suspected [7].

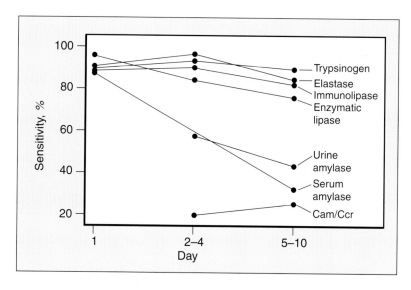

FIGURE 3-9.

Diagnosis of acute pancreatitis. A composite of several studies comparing the sensitivity of diagnostic blood and urine tests in diagnosing acute pancreatitis, depending on the day of presentation to the hospital. On day 1 of abdominal pain, all diagnostic markers are very sensitive. On day 2 and beyond, the serum amylase level drops to normal faster than the lipase of the immunologic markers—immunolipase, tryspinogen, or immuno-elastase. The urinary diagnosis of acute pancreatitis—timed urine amylase collection or the amylase to creatinine clearance ratio (Cam/Ccr)—offers no advantages to the serological diagnosis. (*Adapted from* Steinberg *et al.* [8].)

PROGNOSTIC MARKERS OF SEVERITY

TABLE 3-13. PROGNOSTIC INDICATORS OF SEVERITY

Multiple criteria scales

  Ranson

  Modified Glasgow

  Apache II score

Laboratory parameters—blood/urine

  C reactive protein

  Trypsinogen activation peptide

  Interleukin 6

  Dark fluid on peritoneal tap

Imaging—necrosis/hypoperfusion of computed tomography scan

Clinical parameters—obesity

TABLE 3-13.

Overview of the different prognostic indicators of severity. Multiple criteria lists developed by Dr. John Ranson; the APACHE II score; and clinicians in Glasgow, Scotland are commonly used. Laboratory parameters, such as the serum C reactive protein, are employed in Europe. Imaging with computed tomography is useful in predicting severity if necrosis or fluid collections are present. Recent studies suggest obesity is a risk factor for severe disease.

TABLE 3-14. RANSON CRITERIA FOR SEVERITY OF ACUTE PANCREATITIS

	Non-gallstone pancreatitis (EG, alcohol)	Gallstone pancreatitis
On admission		
Age, y	>55	>70
WBC mm^{-3}	>16,000	>18,000
Blood glucose mg/dL	>200	>220
Serum LDH IU/mL	>350	>400
Serum AST IU/mL	>250	>250
At 48 hours		
Hematocrit ↓ %	>10	>10
BUN ↑ mg/dL	>5	>2
Serum Ca^{++} mg/dL	<8	<8
pO_2 $mmHg$	<60	—
Base deficit mEq/L	>4	>5
Fluid requirements L	>6	>4

TABLE 3-14.

Ranson criteria. There are two lists: one for nongallstone pancreatitis (Ranson 1974) and one for acute gallstone pancreatitis (Ranson 1982). Three or more risk factors are associated with an increased probability of severe disease [9,10].

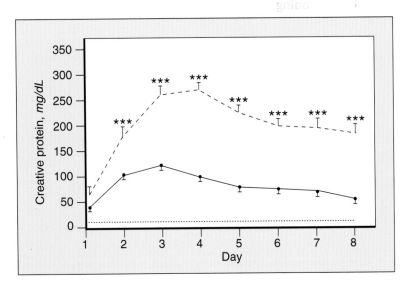

FIGURE 3-10.

Serum C reactive protein (CRP) levels in acute pancreatitis. This test is commonly used in Europe to detect severity of disease. The upper line represents the CRP levels in patients with severe disease, and the middle line represents mild disease. The curves diverge starting on day 2 of the illness. The bottom line represents the upper limit of normal for this test. Asterisks indicate statistical significance from lower curve values. (*Adapted from* Wilson *et al.* [11]; with permission.)

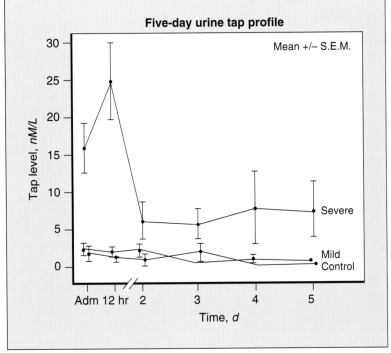

FIGURE 3-11.

Urinary trypsinogen activation peptide (TAP) levels in acute pancreatitis. This is another test that differentiates severe from mild disease according to this study from the United Kingdom. On day 1, there is a clear separation between patients with severe and mild pancreatitis. (*Adapted from* Gudgeon *et al.* [12].)

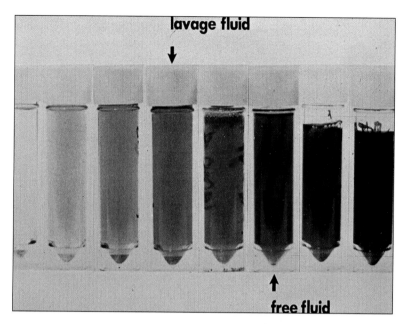

FIGURE 3-12.

Peritoneal aspirates in acute pancreatitis. The color of the peritoneal aspirate of patients with acute pancreatitis can differentiate mild from severe disease. The darker the color (caused by blood, due to hemorrhagic pancreatitis), the greater the severity of the disease is. (*From* McMahon *et al.* [13]; with permission.)

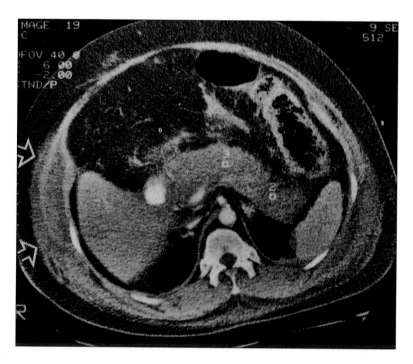

FIGURE 3-13.

Dynamic computed tomography (CT) scan of the pancreas peformed by injecting large doses of intravenous contrast rapidly (bolus injection) and sca   the pancreas with thin cuts. This CT scan shows poor perfusion of the pancreas. The presence of poor perfusion on CT scan has about a 90% predictive value of predicting necrosis at surgery; however, only about 60% of patients with necrosis on CT scan have a severe course clinically [14,15].

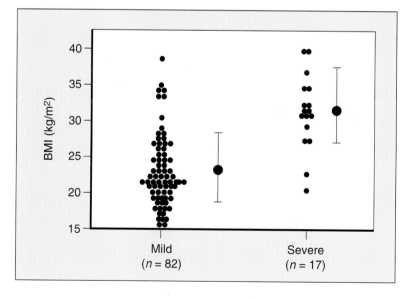

FIGURE 3-14.

This study from South Africa correlates obesity with severity of acute pancreatitis. The horizontal line measures the body mass index (BMI) and represents weight (in kilograms) divided by height (in square meters). Severe disease was more common in obese patients (BMI > 30 kg/m^2) than in nonobese patients. This may be due to the fact that obese patients have more peripancreatic fat that can become necrotic upon release of lipase after initiation of pancreatitis. Bars represent mean ± standard deviation. (*Adapted from* Funnell *et al.* [16]; with permission.)

PROGNOSIS AND COMPLICATIONS

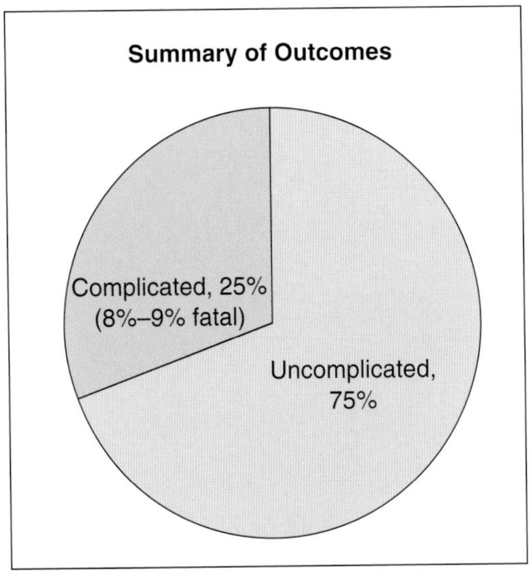

Summary of Outcomes

Complicated, 25% (8%–9% fatal)

Uncomplicated, 75%

FIGURE 3-15.

Overall prognosis of acute pancreatitis taken from the world literature. Approximately 25% of cases are complicated, with a mortality rate of 8% to 9%. Mortality is greater during the first attack than during subsequent attacks.

TABLE 3-15. COMPLICATIONS OF ACUTE PANCREATITIS

Local	Systemic
Necrosis	Shock
Pseudocysts	Respiratory failure
Abcess	Renal failure
Ileus	Metabolic—hypocalcemia, hyperglycemia
Fistulization	Coagulopathy—disseminated intravascular coagulation
Gastrointestinal hemorrhage—pseudoaneurysm	

TABLE 3-15.

Complications of acute pancreatitis can be divided into local and systemic. Complications can also be divided into two groups—early (occurring in the first week, such as pulmonary, renal, and cardiovascular failure) and late (occurring mostly after the first week, such as infected necrosis, pseudocyst, and abscess.)

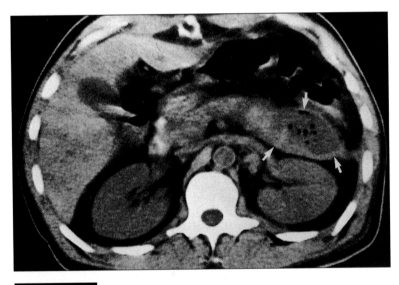

FIGURE 3-16.

A computed tomography (CT) scan of the pancreas indicating gas bubbles within the substance of the pancreas. This suggests pancreatic abscess secondary to gas-producing organisms; however, sterile necrosis with microcommunication with the gut can lead to this CT finding. Only with a fine-needle aspirate can one diagnose an abscess with assurance. (*From* Freeny and Lawson [17]; with permission.)

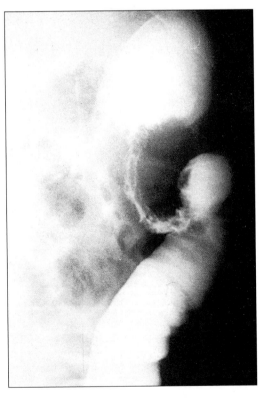

FIGURE 3-17.

An example of colonic obstruction due to pancreatitis. This tends to occur on the left side of the colon. Necrosis and fistulization of the colon can also occur as a late complication. (*From* Huizinga *et al*. [18]; with permission.)

TABLE 3-16. MAJOR CAUSES OF DEATH IN ACUTE PANCREATITIS

Sepsis—infected necrosis/asbscess	Renal
Multiorgan failure	Cardiovascular
Pulmonary (adult respiratory distress syndrome)	Single-organ failure

TABLE 3-16.

The major causes of death in acute pancreatitis are delineated. The two most common causes are infected necrosis and multiorgan failure.

TABLE 3-17. PRINCIPLES OF TREATMENT OF ACUTE PANCREATITIS

Intravascular volume

Analgesia

Put pancreas to "rest"

Nothing by mouth, nasogastric tube only for ileus or vomiting

Treat complications—pulmonary, shock, renal, metabolic

Remove obstructing gallstone in severe gallstone pancreatitis endoscopically

Antibiotics for severe disease

Percutaneous aspiration of pancreas to document infection in patient who fails to respond.

TABLE 3-17.

The principles of treatment of acute pancreatitis are summarized here. Hospitalization is required, and in severe cases, therapy should be administered in an intensive care unit.

TABLE 3-18. EMERGENCY ENDOSCOPIC RETROGRADE CHOLANGIO-PANCREATOGRAPHY PLUS SPHINCTEROTOMY FOR BILIARY PANCREATITIS

121 Patients randomized
59 ERCP + ES
62 conventionally

	ERCP + ES	CONVENTIONAL
Severe (n=53)		
Comp	6/25 (24%)	17/28 (61%)
Mort	1/25 (4%)	5/28 (18%)
Mild (n=68)		
Comp	4/34 (12%)	4/34 (12%)
Mort	0	0

TABLE 3-18.

United Kingdom randomized study comparing emergency endoscopic retrograde cholangiopancreatography (ERCP) (within 72 hours of admission) with endoscopic sphincterotomy (ES) with stone removal versus conventional conservative management in biliary pancreatitis. Results show that complications (Comp) and mortality (Mort) are reduced in the ERCP + ES group in severe gallstone pancreatitis (as defined by the modified Glasgow criteria). In those predicted to have mild disease (by the Glasgow criteria), the ERCP + ES group fared the same as those treated conservatively. (*Adapted from* Neoptolemos *et al.* [19].)

TABLE 3-19. ENDOSCOPIC RETROGRADE CHOLANGIOPANCREATOGRAPHY IN ACUTE GALLSTONE PANCREATITIS

	EMERGENCY	CONSERVATIVE	P VALUE
ALL PATIENTS	N=97	N=98	
Complications	18%	29%	0.07
Mortality	5%	9%	0.400
BILIARY STONE PATIENTS	N=64	N=63	
Complications	16%	33%	0.030
Cholangitis	0%	12%	0.001
Mortality	2%	8%	0.090

TABLE 3-19.

This Hong Kong study randomized 195 patients to emergency endoscopic retrograde cholangiopancreatography (ERCP) within 24 hours of admission versus no emergency ERCP, although most patients in this group received a subsequent ERCP [20]. If a stone was found, it was removed. About two thirds of the total group had gallstones as the etiology. In this subgroup of biliary stone patients, removing gallstones by emergency ERCP reduced complications, especially cholangitis. Mortality was also reduced, but this was not statistically significant. This study and the one summarized in Table 3-18 indicated that it is relatively safe to perform emergency ERCP in acute pancreatitis. Proven utility of ERCP is in the removal of suspected gallstones in patients with severe pancreatitis or in those in whom cholangitis is suspected; however, a more recent study suggests that ERCP may not necessarily improve outcome in biliary pancreatitis [20]. Thus, additional studies are needed to settle this issue.

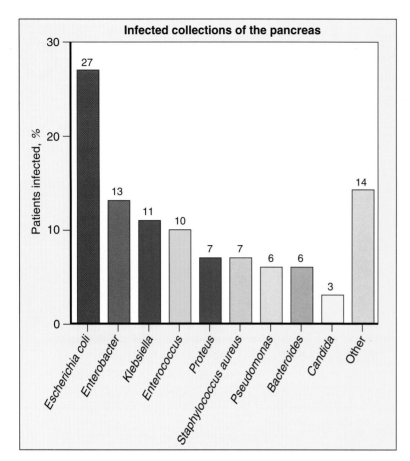

Infected collections of the pancreas

FIGURE 3-18.

Studies in the 1970s using ampicillin showed no effect on the outcome of mild alcoholic pancreatitis; however, this was the wrong group to study (only mild disease), and ampicillin may have been the wrong antibiotic to study. This figure lists the bacteria aspirated from infected pancreatic collections from two large studies. Most of the bacteria are from gram-negative species. The total is greater than 100% because more than one organism may be encountered [21,22].

TABLE 3-20. ANTIBIOTIC THERAPY

Antibiotics with effective penetration
    Ciprofloxacin
    Ofloxacin
    Imipenem
    Metronidazole
Antibiotics with poorer penetration
    Aminoglycosides
    Broad spectrum penicillins
    Third generation cephalosporins

TABLE 3-20.

Studies from Germany show that certain antibiotics (*eg,* ciprofloxacin and imipenem) penetrate necrotic pancreatic and peripancreatic tissues better than others, and achieve bactericidal levels to kill the mostly gram-negative organisms that cause pancreatic infection [23].

TABLE 3-21. IMIPENEM AND NECROTIZING PANCREATITIS

	IMIPENEM	No IMIPENEM	*P*
Pancreatic sepsis	13.0%	30.0%	< 0.01
Nonpancreatic sepsis	14.0%	48%	< 0.01
Death	7.3%	12.1%	Not significant

TABLE 3-21.

In a randomized study from Italy, 74 patients with necrotizing pancreatitis were randomized within 72 hours of admission to receive imipenem 0.5 g/ 7 d (*n*=41) versus no antibiotics (*n*=33). Patients randomized to imipenem had significantly fewer pancreatic and nonpancreatic infections. There was a trend toward lower mortality in the antibiotic group, but it was not statistically significant. This study documents improved outcome in patients with severe pancreatitis who receive a broad-spectrum antibiotic [24].

CONTROVERSIES IN TREATMENT

Dialysis

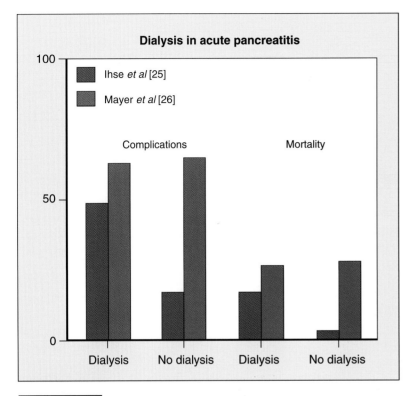

FIGURE 3-19.

Early uncontrolled studies suggested that peritoneal dialysis improved the early complications of acute pancreatitis (pulmonary failure and shock); however, two controlled, randomized European studies have shown no benefit in improving the morbidity and mortality of acute pancreatitis using 2- to 3-day peritoneal dialysis [25,26].

TABLE 3-22. PERITONEAL DIALYSIS (LAVAGE) IN SEVERE PANCREATITIS

PATIENTS	3–4 SIGNS	≥5 SIGNS
Long lavage		
Patients	4	10
Deaths	0	2 (20%)
Abscess	0	3 (30%)
Abscess death	0	0*
Short lavage		
Patients	8	7
Deaths	0	3 (43%)
Abscess	2 (25%)	4 (57%)
Abscess death	0	3 (43%)*

*P = 0.051.

TABLE 3-22.

Ranson and Berman randomized 29 patients with severe pancreatitis to short (2-day) or long (7-day) peritoneal dialysis. He found that those patients who were most ill (≥ 5 Ranson signs) while receiving long dialysis had fewer pancreatic abscesses and fewer deaths from abscess. Peritoneal dialysis in severe pancreatitis remains a controversial issue [27].

SURGERY

TABLE 3-23. ROLE OF SURGERY

Débride necrosis
   Infected/? sterile

Drain abscess/pseudocyst

When diagnosis is in doubt
   Perforated viscus
   Small bowel obstruction/infarction

TABLE 3-23.

The current indications for surgery in acute pancreatitis are delineated here. The timing and the role of surgical débridement in sterile and infected pancreatic necrosis is debated.

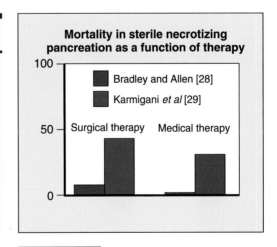

FIGURE 3-20.

There are no controlled studies comparing surgical débridement versus medical management either for sterile or infected necrosis. Two retrospective analyses showed no benefit in mortality in those patients receiving surgical débridement for sterile pancreatic necrosis versus those who received medical management [28,29].

TABLE 3-24. DIFFERENTIATING INFECTED FROM STERILE NECROSIS

Fever curve and white blood count not predictive

Infected patients have greater number of multiorgan failures (cardiovascular, renal, pulmonary, gastrointestinal bleeding)

Infected patients have more necrosis on computed tomography scan

Fine-needle aspiration is required

TABLE 3-24.

Sterile necrosis cannot be differentiated easily from infected necrosis by clinical criteria. A few guidelines (clues) are listed here. Fine needle aspiration of the pancreas is needed to differentiate the two entities.

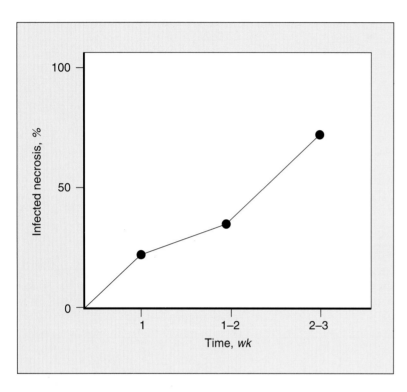

FIGURE 3-21.

Infected necrosis can occur within the first week of illness, but tends to occur more frequently during the second and third weeks. The natural history of infected necrosis is unknown. Although there are some cases of survival with antibiotic treatment alone, patients with documented pancreatic infection are usually treated with surgical débridement. Percutaneous drainage of infected fluid collections can sometimes temporize the need for emergency surgery. (*Adapted from* Beger *et al.* [21].)

REFERENCES

1. Venu RP, Greenen JE, Hogan W, *et al.*: Idiopathic recurrent pancreatitis: An approach to diagnosis and treatment. *Dig Dis Sci* 1989, 34:56–60.

2. Lee SP, Nicholls JF, *et al.*: Biliary sludge as a cause of acute pancreatitis. *N Engl J Med* 1992, 326:589–593.

3. Ros E, Navarro S, Bru C, *et al.*: Occult microlithiasis in "idiopathic pancreatitis": Prevention of relapses by cholecystectomy or ursodeoxycholic acid therapy. *Gastroenterology* 1991, 101:1701–1709.

4. Steinberg WM, Tenner S: Acute pancreatitis. *N Engl J Med* 1994, 330:1198–1210.

5. Czernobilsky B, Mikat K: The diagnostic significance of interstitial pancreatitis found at autopsy. *Am J Clin Pathol* 1964, 41:35.

6. Klatt EC: Pathology of pentamidine-induced pancreatitis. *Arch Pathol Lab Med* 1992, 116:162–164.

7. Neoptolemos JP, Hall AW, Finlay DW, *et al.*: The urgent diagnosis of gallstones in acute pancreatitis: A prospective study of three methods. *Br J Surg* 1984, 71:230–233.

8. Steinberg WM, Goldstein SS, Davis ND, *et al.*: Diagnostic assays in acute pancreatitis. *Ann Intern Med* 1985, 102:576–580.

9. Ranson JHC, Rifkind KM, Turner JW: Prognostic signs and nonoperative lavage in acute pancreatitis. *Surg Gynecol Obstet* 1976, 143:209–213.

10. Ranson JHC: Etiological and prognostic factors in human acute pancreatitis. *Am J Gastroenterol* 1982, 77:177–181.

11. Wilson C, Heads A, Shenkin A, *et al.*: C-reactive protein, antiproteases and complement as objective markers in acute pancreatitis. *Br J Surg* 1989, 76: 177–181.

12. Gudgeon AM, Heath DI, Hurley P, *et al.*: Trypsinogen activation peptides assay in the early prediction of severity of acute pancreatitis. *Lancet* 1990, 335:4–8.

13. McMahon MJ, Playforth M, Pickford I: A comparative study of methods for the prediction of severity of acute pancreatitis. *Br J Surg* 1980, 67:22.

14. Bradley EL, Murphy F, Ferguson C: Prediction of pancreatic necrosis by dynamic pancreatography. *Ann Surg* 1990, 210:495–504.

15. London NJM, Lesse T, Lavelle JM: Rapid bolus contrast enhanced dynamic computed tomography in acute pancreatitis: A prospective study. *Br J Surg* 1991, 78:1452–1456.

16. Funnell IC, Bormann PC, Weakley SP, *et al.*: Obesity: An important prognostic factor in acute pancreatitis. *Br J Surg* 1993, 80:484–486.

17. Freeny PC, Lawson TL: *Radiology of the Pancreas.* New York: Springer-Verlag; 1982: 306–398.

18. Huizinga WK, Reddy E, Simjee AE: Pancreatitis and large bowel obstruction. *Dig Dis Sci* 1987, 32:108–109.

19. Neoptolemos JP, Carr-Locke D, James D, *et al.*: Controlled trial of urgent endoscopic retrograde cholangiopancreatography and endoscopic sphincterotomy versus conservative treatment for acute pancreatitis due to gallstones. *Lancet* 1988, 2:979–983.

20. Fan ST, Lai ECS, Mok FPT, *et al.*: Early treatment of acute biliary pancreatitis by endoscopic papillotomy. *N Engl J Med* 1993, 328:228–232.

21. Beger HG, Bittner R, Block S, *et al.*: Bacterial contamination of pancreatic necrosis: A prospective clinical study. *Gastroenterology* 1986, 91:433–438.

22. Gerzof SG, Banks PA, Robbins AH, *et al.*: Early diagnosis of pancreatic infection by computed tomography-guided aspiration. *Gastroenterology* 1987, 93:1315–1320.

23. Buchler M, Malfertheiner P, Fries H, *et al.*: Human pancreatic tissue concentration of bactericidal antibiotics. *Gastroenterology* 1992, 103:1902–1908.

24. Pederzoli P, Bassi C, Vesentini S, *et al.*: A randomized multicenter clinical trial of antibiotic prophylaxis of septic complications in acute necrotizing pancreatitis with imipenem. *Surg Gynecol Obstet* 1993, 176:480–483.

25. Ihse I, Evander A, Holmberg JT, *et al.*: Influence of peritoneal lavage on objective prognostic signs in acute pancreatitis. *Ann Surg* 1986, 204:122–127.

26. Mayer AD, McMahon MJ, Corfield AP, *et al.*: Controlled clinical trial of peritoneal lavage for the treatment of severe acute pancreatitis. *N Engl J Med* 1985, 312:399–404.

27. Ranson JHC, Berman RS: Long peritoneal lavage decreases pancreatic sepsis in acute pancreatitis. *Ann Surg* 1990, 211:708–710.

28. Bradley EL, Allen K: A prospective longitudinal study of observation versus surgical intervention in the management of necrotizing pancreatitis. *Am J Surg* 1991, 161:19–24.

29. Karmigani I, Porter KA, Langevin RE, Banks PA: Prognostic factors in sterile pancreatic necrosis. *Gastroenterology* 1992, 103:1636–1640.

Chapter 4

Chronic Pancreatitis

Chronic pancreatitis is a disease process characterized by irreversible damage to the pancreas, as distinct from the reversible changes as seen in acute pancreatitis. The condition is best defined by the presence of histologic abnormalities, including chronic inflammation, fibrosis, and progressive destruction of both exocrine, and eventually, endocrine tissue. In most patients, pancreatic tissue is not available for evaluation, so that other clinical features and diagnostic tests are used to define the disease process. Many circumstances cause chronic pancreatitis, but all lead ultimately to irreversible morphologic damage to the pancreas, and they can produce the cardinal complications of chronic pancreatitis: abdominal pain, steatorrhea, and diabetes mellitus. Long-term alcohol abuse is the most common cause of chronic pancreatitis, but other important causes include obstruction of the main pancreatic duct, hyperlipidemia, and idiopathic forms, which may account for up to 25% of cases. The natural history of chronic pancreatitis is one of progressive destruction of the gland occurring over 10 to 20 years, but the natural histories of alcoholic and idiopathic chronic pancreatitis are substantially different.

Abdominal pain, the most common symptom of chronic pancreatitis, has a variety of underlying causes. Exocrine insufficiency (steatorrhea) and endocrine insufficiency (diabetes mellitus) occur less commonly than abdominal pain, and are markers of substantial destruction of the gland, and hence a far advanced disease process. The diagnosis of chronic pancreatitis is relatively easy in patients with severe, advanced disease. These patients usually have a long history of compatible symptoms, steatorrhea with or without diabetes, and readily identifiable damage to the pancreas visible on imaging studies (*eg*, diffuse calcification of the gland, marked dilation of the pancreatic duct, pseudocysts). Although the diagnosis is

CHRIS E. FORSMARK
PHILLIP P. TOSKES

usually straightforward in such patients with "big-duct" disease, the diagnostic evaluation of patients with less advanced disease and with relatively normal results from imaging studies is much more challenging. These patients with "small-duct" disease are more common than is usually appreciated by clinicians; therefore, diagnosis requires the use of sensitive tests of pancreatic function.

Treatment of patients begins with the recognition of complications that require specific therapy, such as duodenal or biliary obstruction or a symptomatic pseudocyst. Cessation of alcohol consumption, treatment of malnutrition and steatorrhea, and therapy with analgesics are useful initial steps. Medical therapy for chronic pain may also include agents that reduce excessive feedback stimulation of the pancreas, in particular, nonenteric-coated pancreatic enzyme supplements. Patients with big-duct disease who fail medical therapy are candidates for surgical duct decompression. In patients with refractory disease, pancreatic resection or experimental therapies to reduce pancreatic feedback stimulation may also be considered.

■ CLASSIFICATION OF CHRONIC PANCREATITIS

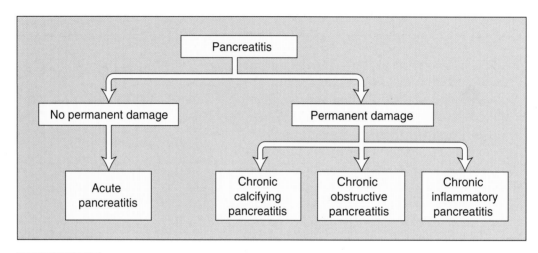

FIGURE 4-1.

Marseilles-Rome classification. The tremendous variability of symptoms and diversity of etiologies have made classification of chronic pancreatitis difficult, and a variety of systems have been developed to classify chronic pancreatitis. The most recent international symposium [1], in 1988, defined three forms of chronic pancreatitis based on morphologic criteria: chronic calcifying pancreatitis, chronic obstructive pancreatitis, and chronic inflammatory pancreatitis. Chronic calcifying pancreatitis is defined by the presence of calcified stones within the pancreatic ductal system, and usually results from long-standing alcohol abuse. Chronic obstructive pancreatitis is defined as downstream obstruction of the main pancreatic duct with upstream dilation; stones are infrequently seen with this condition. Chronic inflammatory pancreatitis is defined by a relative lack of either calcification or dilation of the main pancreatic duct. This classification system is not useful in most clinical situations.

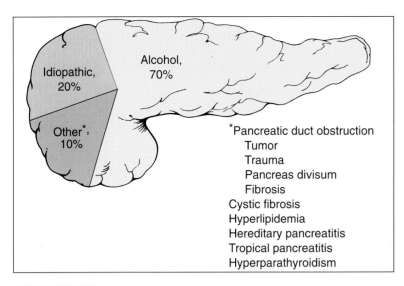

FIGURE 4-2.

Classification by etiology. Chronic pancreatitis may also be classified by its presumed cause. Chronic alcoholism accounts for approximately 70% of all cases of chronic pancreatitis. Prolonged and substantial abuse is generally required to produce chronic pancreatitis, and most (but not all) patients who present with an episode of acute pancreatitis caused by alcohol consumption already have chronic pancreatic damage. Chronic obstruction of the pancreatic duct may also produce chronic pancreatitis, such as that caused by tumors, trauma, pseudocysts, inflammation and fibrosis (such as after a severe episode of acute pancreatitis), pancreas divisum (with associated minor papilla stenosis), and even after prolonged endoscopic stenting of the the pancreatic duct. After traumatic injury to the pancreatic duct (such as after a motor vehicle accident or a stab wound), chronic pancreatitis may develop within a few months. Pancreas divisum commonly occurs as a normal variant (in 10% of the population), and most patients remain asymptomatic. This variant occurs after nonfusion of the two pancreatic buds during development, so that most pancreatic secretion in the dorsal segment drains through the minor papilla rather than the major papilla. A small subset of patients have both pancreas divisum and obstruction at the minor papilla, which may produce both acute relapsing pancreatitis or, more rarely, chronic obstructive pancreatitis. Hyperlipidemia, particularly when the serum triglycerides are above 1000 mg/dL, may produce both acute and chronic pancreatitis. Tropical chronic pancreatitis, probably caused by malnutrition and toxic products in the diet, is rare in the United States. Cystic fibrosis is an important cause of chronic pancreatitis in children, although with improved pulmonary care these patients may live to adulthood. Despite careful evaluation, about 20% of patients (in some studies as high as 30%) have no specific identifiable etiology, and are thus classified as having idiopathic chronic pancreatitis.

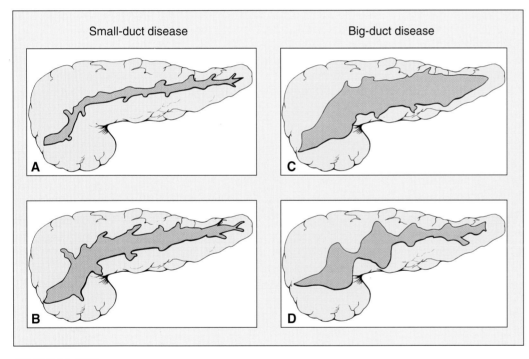

FIGURE 4-3.

Classification by pancreatic duct morphology. The abnormalities demonstrated in the pancreatic duct by endoscopic retrograde pancreatography (ERP) or inferred by findings using computed tomography are the most clinically useful means to classify chronic pancreatitis. This system divides patients into two major groups: big-duct disease, characterized by substantial abnormalities of the main pancreatic duct (particularly dilation, intraductal stones, and strictures), and small-duct disease (or chronic pancreatitis with minimal change), where abnormalities of the main pancreatic duct are absent and changes are limited to the smaller side branches of the duct or the pancreatic parenchyma. In general, patients with big-duct disease have more advanced chronic pancreatitis, often with associated exocrine and endocrine insufficiency (steatorrhea and diabetes mellitus), and commonly have alcoholic chronic pancreatitis. Patients with small-duct disease tend to have less advanced disease and more commonly have idiopathic chronic pancreatitis or early stages of alcoholic chronic pancreatitis. The distinction between these two groups of patients is usually straightforward after the diagnosis of chronic pancreatitis is made; the distinction carries significant therapeutic implications (*see* section on Treatment). **A–B**, examples of small-duct disease are presented. **A**, A nondilated main pancreatic duct with clubbing and dilation of the side branches; **B**, a mildly dilated main duct with abnormal side branches. **C–D**, changes of big-duct disease. **C**, Markedly dilated main pancreatic duct; **D**, end-stage "chain-of-lakes" appearance.

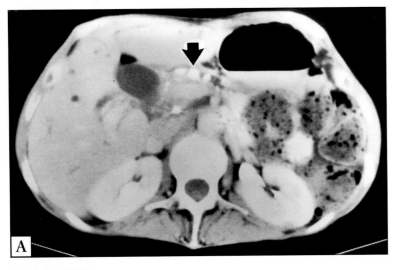

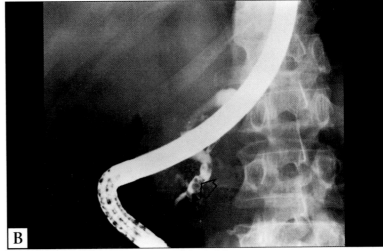

FIGURE 4-4.

Pathophysiology. The specific mechanism by which alcohol produces chronic pancreatitis is unknown, but it does appear to require substantial alcohol ingestion over at least 6 to 12 years. Various physiologic abnormalities have been documented in both animal models and in humans, including a direct toxic effect of pancreatic acinar cells, stimulation of pancreatic secretion, interference with normal intracellular protein trafficking, and the promotion of the formation of protein plugs within the ductal system. These plugs often become calcified, producing pancreatic ductal stones. Whether these stones contribute to the pathogenesis of alcoholic chronic pancreatitis by obstructing the pancreatic ducts is unknown. They may merely be a marker of alcoholic chronic

pancreatitis rather than its cause. A, Multiple calcified stones within the pancreatic duct on a computed tomography scan (arrow). B, A stone within the main pancreatic duct at endoscopic retrograde pancreatography (filling defect within the dye column in the main pancreatic duct [arrow]).

The specific mechanism by which other causes of chronic pancreatitis produce pancreatic injury is also unknown. For example, it is unclear if conditions that obstruct the pancreatic duct produce damage by mere obstruction or if additional insults (such as low-grade infection, activation of pancreatic digestive enzymes, inflammation, or high pressure within the obstructed duct) are required.

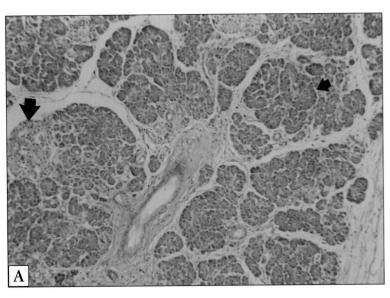

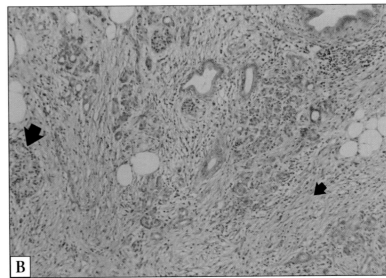

FIGURE 4-5.

Histology. Regardless of the specific cause of chronic pancreatitis, the histologic result is similar. Pancreatic inflammation, together with progressive fibrosis, leads to destruction of the acinar cells either focally or diffusely, producing exocrine insufficiency and steatorrhea. Intraductal concretions and stones may form, which may block the flow of pancreatic secretions and augment the damage. Inflammation involving pancreatic nerves is also

commonly found. The endocrine tissue (the islets of Langerhans) is typically spared until late in the disease process, making diabetes mellitus a late complication. A, Normal pancreatic tissue is demonstrated with a normal acinar architecture (small arrow) and islets of Langerhans (large arrow). B, Changes of chronic pancreatitis include destruction of acinar tissue with replacement by fibrosis (small arrow), but the islets remain intact (large arrow).

CLINICAL FEATURES

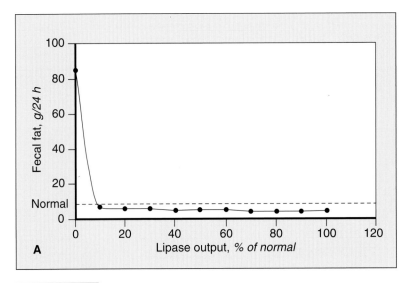

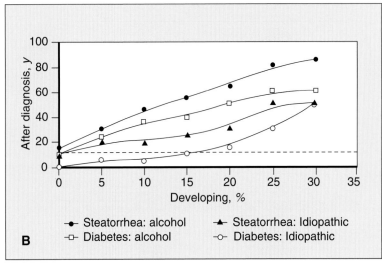

FIGURE 4-6.

Steatorrhea and diabetes mellitus. Malabsorption and weight loss are markers of more advanced chronic pancreatitis. The pancreas has substantial reserve, and malabsorption is not typically seen until 90% of pancreatic exocrine secretion has been lost [2]. **A,** The degree of damage necessary for the development of steatorrhea. In addition, patients may lose weight because they avoid food or may have an inadequate nutritional intake caused by chronic alcoholism. Fat and protein are more poorly absorbed than carbohydrates in patients with chronic pancreatitis. Despite often substantial steatorrhea, specific deficiencies of fat-soluble vitamins is unusual. Likewise, despite measurable malabsorption of vitamins (including vitamin B_{12}), specific deficiencies are unusual unless chronic alcoholism and inadequate vitamin intake are present.

Endocrine insufficiency (diabetes mellitus) is an even later occurrence than exocrine insufficiency. Up to 60% to 70% of patients with alcoholic pancreatitis may ultimately develop diabetes mellitus after 20 years of disease, at which time most will have diffuse pancreatic calcifications [3,4]. **B,** Patients with idiopathic chronic pancreatitis develop steatorrhea and diabetes mellitus at a slower rate than patients with alcoholic chronic pancreatitis. Ketoacidosis is unusual, but frequent treatment-associated episodes of hypoglycemia may be a problem. Complications of diabetes mellitus, such as neuropathy and retinopathy, occur as frequently as in other forms of diabetes if incidence is corrected for disease duration. (**A,** *Adapted from* Dimagno *et al.* [2]; with permission. **B,** *Adapted from* Layer *et al.* [4].)

DIAGNOSIS

TABLE 4-1. DIAGNOSTIC TESTS

FUNCTION	STRUCTURE
Direct hormonal stimulation tests	Endoscopic retrograde pancreatography
Bentiromide test	Computed tomography
Serum trypsin-like immunoreactivity	Endoscopic ultrasound
Fecal chymotrypsin or fecal elastase	Magnetic resonance imaging
Quantitative fecal fat	Ultrasonography
Blood glucose	Plain abdominal radiograph

Tests are listed in order of decreasing sensitivity.

TABLE 4-1.

Diagnostic tests. The diagnosis of chronic pancreatitis is most reliably based on the demonstration of consistent histologic abnormalities, but pancreatic tissue is difficult and risky to obtain, and therefore is not available in most patients. Commonly used diagnostic tests rely on abnormalities of either morphology or function. The available diagnostic tests are listed in this table in order of decreasing sensitivity. As chronic pancreatitis progresses, obvious abnormalities develop that make diagnosis straightforward, such as diffuse pancreatic calcifications, a markedly dilated duct, and complications such as a pseudocyst, steatorrhea, and diabetes. Most tests will provide a diagnosis in patients with this far-advanced disease; however, only the most sensitive tests have the potential of identifying the large group of patients with less-advanced disease states.

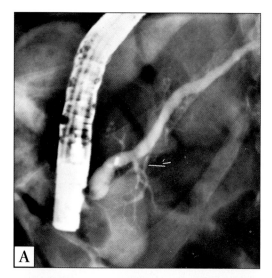

A

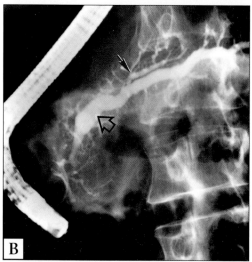

B

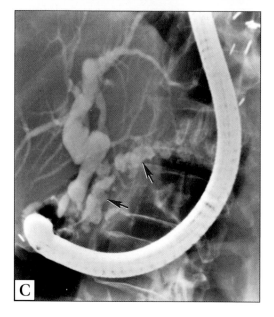

C

FIGURE 4-7.

Tests of structure: endoscopic retrograde pancreatography (ERP). The most sensitive diagnostic test for chronic pancreatitis that relies on structural changes is ERP. The diagnosis of chronic pancreatitis is based on changes in both the main pancreatic duct and the side branches. The Cambridge criteria [5] define those changes in the main duct suggestive of chronic pancreatitis as dilation, narrowing or stricture formation, irregular contour, associated filling of cavities or pseudocysts, or filling defects (pancreatic duct stones). Side-branch changes include shortening, dilation, and clubbing. At its most advanced stages, the "chain-of-lakes" appearance of alternate dilation and strictures is characteristic of chronic pancreatitis. In advanced chronic pancreatitis these marked changes in the main pancreatic duct (big-duct disease) are common; therefore, ERP is an extremely accurate test. In less advanced disease (small-duct disease), however, the changes are often inadequate to be diagnostic of chronic pancreatitis [6]. **A**, Mild changes with minimal dilation of the pancreatic duct and clubbing of the side branches (*arrow*). **B**, More advanced changes with moderate dilation of the main duct (*large arrow*) and coexistent changes in the side branches (*small arrow*). **C**, Advanced disease, with a characteristic "chain-of-lakes" appearance of the pancreatic duct (*arrows*). Substantial evidence now exists that a significant proportion of patients with histologically proven chronic pancreatitis will have normal or only minimally abnormal results of pancreatograms [7,8]. In addition, various other conditions may mimic the pancreatographic changes of chronic pancreatitis, including normal aging, a recent attack of acute pancreatitis, pancreatic carcinoma, and findings after pancreatic duct stenting [6]. The reported sensitivity of ERP for chronic pancreatitis is 67% to 93%, with specificities ranging from 89% to 100% [9]. These results are generated from studies evaluating patients with more advanced disease, so they are clearly overestimates of true sensitivity and specificity. ERP may also be used to develop therapeutic rather than diagnostic information. In particular, ERP can document main-duct dilation, which is a prerequisite for consideration of surgical duct decompression (Puestow's procedure). ERP can also be useful in differentiating pancreatic malignancy from chronic pancreatitis, both by morphologic criteria and by obtaining cytology from pancreatic duct strictures.

In addition to the abnormalities already described, ERP may document pancreas divisum. This variant anatomy, wherein the bulk of pancreatic secretion drains through the minor papilla, occurs in 10% of the population; in the vast majority of patients, it does not lead to pancreatic disease. In a small minority of patients, obstruction to flow at the minor papilla may produce either acute pancreatitis or chronic pancreatitis. This can be definitively established if the dorsal ductal system is dilated or has changes of chronic pancreatitis, or if a hormonal stimulation test (discussed later) is abnormal. In the absence of these diagnostic criteria, it should not be assumed that this variant is producing the chronic abdominal pain.

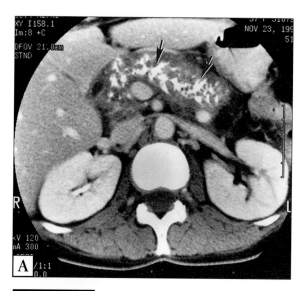
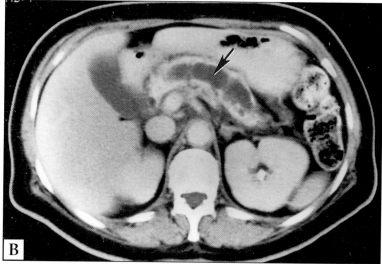

Tests of structure: Computed tomography (CT). Findings on CT that suggest chronic pancreatitis include diffuse calcification, ductal dilation, gland atrophy, irregular contour, and associated pseudocysts [9]. CT is less accurate than endoscopic retrograde pancreatography for the diagnosis of chronic pancreatitis, although the new spiral CT technology allows improved resolution of small structures, such as the pancreatic duct, and appears more accurate than earlier scanning methods. **A**, Diffuse pancreatic calcification (*arrows*). **B**, Markedly dilated pancreatic duct (*arrow*) with atrophy of the pancreas. MR imaging has not been evaluated systematically, although the newer "turboflash" technology and use of oral contrast agents has markedly improved the image quality of scans of the pancreas.

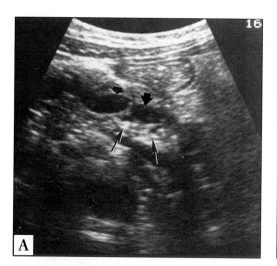
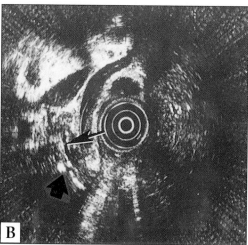

Tests of structure: ultrasonography. Ultrasound is an inexpensive, noninvasive diagnostic test that does not submit the patient to ionizing radiation. It is limited by its poor sensitivity (60%–70%) and inability to image the pancreas in the presence of overlying intestinal gas. Characteristic ultrasound findings include gland atrophy, diffuse calcifications, dilation of the pancreatic duct, and an increase in echogenicity with a heterogeneous pattern [9]. Conversely, ultrasound is quite useful in the detection of pancreatic pseudocysts. **A**, Pancreatic calcifications on conventional ultrasonography (*thin arrows*) and a dilated, segmented pancreatic duct (*thick arrows*). Endoscopic ultrasonography has only begun to be evaluated for use in chronic pancreatitis, but early results are promising. **B**, Endosonographic image of the body of the pancreas with a visible pancreatic duct (*thin arrow*) and calcifications within the gland (*thick arrow*). The circular target structure in the center is the instrument.

Tests of structure: plain abdominal radiograph. The finding of diffuse pancreatic calcification is a specific marker of chronic pancreatitis, but it is only seen in far-advanced disease. Focal calcification is not diagnostic of chronic pancreatitis, and may be seen in a number of other diseases. Although patients with alcoholic chronic pancreatitis will commonly develop diffuse calcifications (70% of patients after 15 years of observation), patients with idiopathic pancreatitis do so only rarely (20%–40% after 15 years of follow-up) [4]. The low sensitivity of plain radiographic limits their use as a diagnostic tool. This figure demonstrates diffuse pancreatic calcification (*arrows*).

TABLE 4-2. HORMONAL STIMULATION TESTS FOR CHRONIC PANCREATITIS

DIAGNOSTIC TEST	SENSITIVITY, %	SPECIFICITY, %	COST*, $
Hormonal (secretin) stimulation test	90+	90+	637
Computed tomography	70–80	70–80	895
Endoscopic retrograde cholangiopancreatography	70–80	80	1709
Serum trypsin	50	90	160

*Cost calculated at University of Florida, 1994.

TABLE 4-2.

Tests of function: hormonal stimulation tests for chronic pancreatitis. The function of the pancreas can be measured directly by stimulating secretion with a secretagogue (secretin or secretin plus cholecystokinin) and collecting pancreatic secretions by an oroduodenal tube. The sensitivity of these tests may be as high as 90% or greater, with a specificity of 90% [6,9]. Direct hormonal stimulation tests are more sensitive, more accurate, and better able to diagnose chronic pancreatitis in its less severe forms than any other diagnostic test for chronic pancreatitis. This table compares commonly used diagnostic tests for chronic pancreatitis. Studies comparing diagnostic tests for chronic pancreatitis have also documented patients with normal tests of structure (endoscopic retrograde pancreatography and computed tomography), but also abnormalities of pancreatic function. Two other investigations have confirmed the presence of chronic pancreatitis in some of these patients based on pancreatic biopsy, confirming the existence of this important subset of patients with small-duct disease or "minimal-change" chronic pancreatitis [7,8]. In patients with less advanced disease, direct hormonal stimulation tests remain the only means to confirm the presence of chronic pancreatitis. Despite their accuracy and safety, direct hormonal stimulation tests are only done at a few institutions.

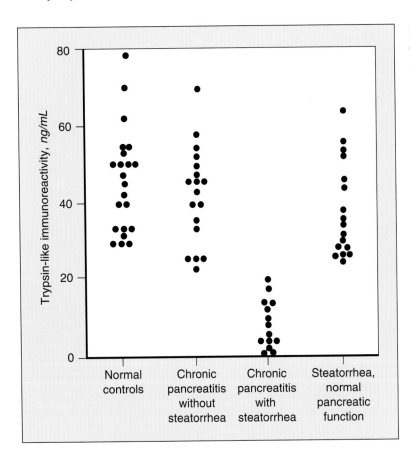

FIGURE 4-11.

Tests of function: simple markers. The most useful simple marker for chronic pancreatitis is serum trypsin-like immunoreactivity (serum trypsin level). Very low levels of trypsin (< 20 ng/mL) are relatively specific for chronic pancreatitis, although ductal obstruction (eg, from pancreatic carcinoma) may also produce these low levels. The test is accurate in patients with more advanced chronic pancreatitis (ie, in the presence of steatorrhea), but is insensitive in less advanced disease [10]. This figure demonstrates the utility of this test in advanced chronic pancreatitis.

The measurement of fecal chymotrypsin also appears to diagnose patients with advanced disease accurately, but is unable to detect chronic pancreatitis in the absence of steatorrhea. It is more cumbersome to use than serum trypsin and has no advantages to recommend it. Fecal elastase may be more sensitive, but further work is needed. The measurement of 72-hour fecal fat to document malabsorption of serum glucose to document endocrine insufficiency may be important in the management of patients with chronic pancreatitis; however, such tests are too insensitive to be used as diagnostic tests. (*Adapted from* Jacobson *et al.* [10]; with permission.)

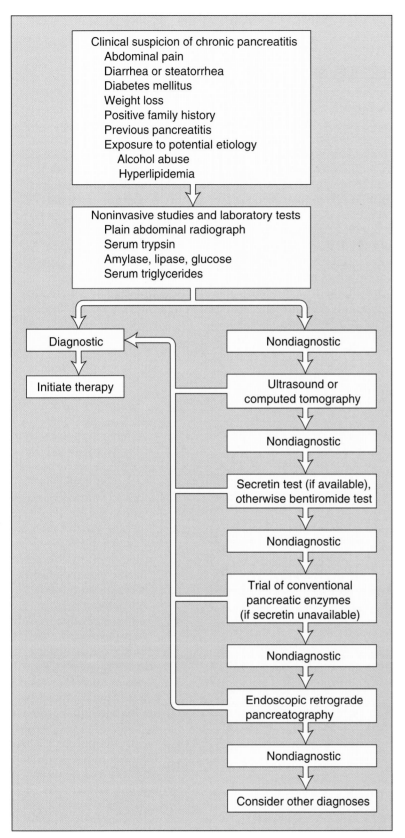

FIGURE 4-12.

Strategy for diagnosis. The overall diagnostic strategy should take into account the relative accuracy, cost, and risks of each diagnostic test. In its advanced form, chronic pancreatitis can be confirmed by a variety of diagnostic tests, so that overall cost and risk of diagnostic tests should be the major concern. In patients with less advanced disease, the accuracy, and in particular, the sensitivity of the diagnostic test become more important. All of this must be tempered by the availability of the variety of diagnostic tests, in particular, the fact that direct hormonal stimulation tests are not universally available. In centers where direct hormonal stimulation tests are not available, a trial of conventional (*ie*, nonenteric-coated) pancreatic enzymes should be considered as a therapeutic trail in patients without major abnormalities of the pancreatic duct because all other diagnostic tests are less sensitive. (*See* section on Treatment for a discussion of the use of enzymes to treat pain.)

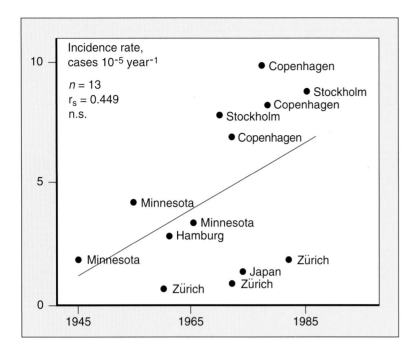

FIGURE 4-13.

Incidence and prevalence. The only prospective study to evaluate the incidence and prevalence of chronic pancreatitis was performed in Copenhagen. It noted an incidence of 8.2 new cases per 100,000 population per year and a prevalence of 27.4 cases per 100,000 population [11]. A number of other studies [12] have estimated incidence of less than 2 per 100,000 population to 10 per 100,000 population. Although it might seem these discrepancies could be explained by the rate of alcohol consumption in the population studied, this does not appear to be the case. All these studies are flawed in that they only identify the patients with more advanced disease or those who have sought medical attention. A substantial number of patients with less advanced disease (small-duct disease) and less severe symptoms were obviously not counted; the true incidence and prevalence of chronic pancreatitis is probably substantially higher than these studies would suggest. (*Adapted from* Worning [12].)

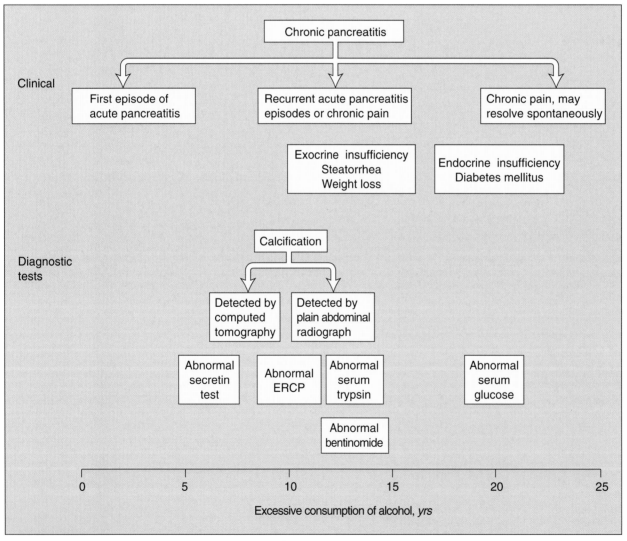

FIGURE 4-14.

Natural history. The natural history of chronic pancreatitis is one of progressive destruction of exocrine and endocrine tissue. The condition of patients with alcoholic pancreatitis appears to deteriorate faster than that of patients with idiopathic pancreatitis [4,13]. Some studies have estimated exocrine insufficiency may develop in 80% of patients with alcoholic chronic pancreatitis after 4 years of follow-up, and endocrine insufficiency in up to 70% after 6 years of follow-up.

One natural history study [4] suggested these estimates may be too high, demonstrating a median time to exocrine insufficiency of 13.1 years (60% of patients after 15 years of follow-up) in patients with alcoholic chronic pancreatitis. In this same study, patients with early-onset idiopathic chronic pancreatitis rarely developed exocrine insufficiency (median time 26.3 years, 25% at 15 years of follow-up), and endocrine insufficiency even more rarely (median time 27.5 years, 10% at 15 years of follow-up). This figure shows an estimated evolution of alcoholic chronic pancreatitis.

Chronic pancreatitis is a disease that is most often managed on an outpatient basis. In 1987, 122,000 office visits were made [14]. During this same time, 20,300 patients were admitted to hospitals with a first-listed diagnosis of chronic pancreatitis whereas 56,200 were admitted with chronic pancreatitis included as one of the diagnoses [14].

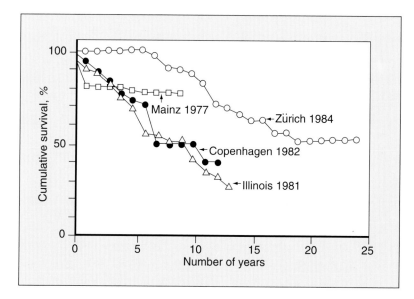

Figure 4-15.

Mortality. The mortality rate associated with the diagnosis of chronic pancreatitis can be substantial, with series reporting 20% to 60% 10-year mortality [12]. Most deaths are not caused by chronic pancreatitis. About 20% of all deaths can be attributed directly to chronic pancreatitis and its complications, with the remaining deaths resulting from cardiovascular disease, extrapancreatic malignancies, chronic alcoholism and its complications, and pancreatic carcinoma [14]. Shown here are cumulative survival curves from four studies of patients with chronic pancreatitis patients who almost exclusively had alcoholism. (*Adapted from* Worning [12]; with permission.)

▌TREATMENT

TABLE 4-3. TREATMENT OF PAIN

Remove inciting process

  Discontinue consumption of alcohol

  Treat hyperlipidemia

Treat complications

  Pseudocyst

  Duodenal obstruction

  Common bile duct obstruction

Analgesics

  Non-narcotic

  Narcotic

Suppress pancreatic secretion

  Pancreatic enzymes

  Investigational agents

Modify neural transmission

  Celiac plexus block

Relieve pancreatic ductal obstruction

  Endoscopic stents (?)

  Surgery

Remove pancreas through partial or complete surgery

Table 4-3.

Treatment of pain, an overview. The available treatment strategies are outlined in this table. Cessation of consumption of alcohol is a prudent step in patients with alcoholic chronic pancreatitis, but the effect on pancreatic damage is quite variable. Although stopping alcohol consumption may allow for recovery of some pancreatic function, in many patients the disease progresses despite sobriety, albeit possibly at a slower pace. Analgesics are usually required, and many patients require narcotics. The risk of addiction to such drugs is present, and is a particular problem in patients with a history of addictive behavior (chronic alcoholism or drug abuse) and in patients with little social support. Despite the risk of addiction (< 20% overall), adequate pain control should be the primary concern.

  Treatments that reduce pancreatic secretion may relieve pain by reducing pancreatic pressure or by other as yet unknown mechanisms. These form the basis for medical therapy of pain, and are discussed in detail in the following figures. Attempts to block neural transmission by celiac axis block are generally ineffective in chronic pancreatitis or are of only short-lived duration, making this technique of little utility for the long-term management of these patients. The effectiveness of surgical therapy in selected patients is discussed in subsequent figures.

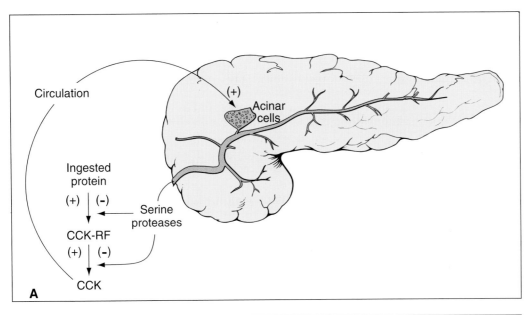

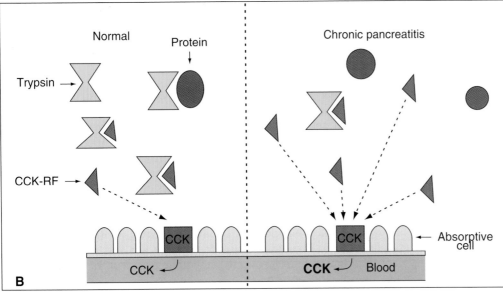

meal. Several of these enzymes (the serine proteases, trypsin, chymotrypsin, and elastase) digest protein, but are also able to digest CCK-RF. When most ingested protein has been digested, excess serine proteases remain and digest the remaining CCK-RF. This feedback system, therefore, stimulates pancreatic secretion when it is needed after eating and stops pancreatic secretion after the meal has been digested. A slow delivery of serine proteases to the duodenum between meals keeps CCK-RF at low levels. In patients with chronic pancreatitis, delivery of digestive enzymes to the duodenum is inadequate, so that CCK-RF escapes destruction and is present at high levels. **B,** The duodenal lumen. On the left side, under normal conditions, CCK-RF is digested by trypsin (and other serine proteases), and is present in low concentrations, leading to a low basal secretion of CCK. On the right side, serine proteases in chronic pancreatitis are present in inadequate quantity to digest CCK-RF, which leads to marked stimulation of CCK release and high levels of CCK in the blood. This high level of CCK, in turn, leads to continuous hyperstimulation of the pancreas, which produces pain by increasing pancreatic pressure or by some as yet unknown mechanism. Treatments that replace the missing enzymes or in some other way reduce CCK levels should therefore help relieve pain.

Several important points need to be kept in mind about manipulating this feedback system for therapeutic benefit: (1) only the duodenum is involved in the feedback loop; exogenous enzyme therapy for pain must therefore be formulated to release enzymes in the duodenum (and the duodenum must be exposed to these enzymes; in patients with a Billroth-II gastrectomy, the duodenum is not exposed to the food stream and enzymes would be ineffective); (2) only the serine proteases, trypsin, chymotrypsin, and elastase, are active in destroying CCK-RF; and (3) not all patients with chronic pancreatitis have pain based on a disorder of this normal feedback loop. (David C. Whitcomb, Personal communication.)

FIGURE 4-16.

Theoretical basis for pain relief by reducing pancreatic secretion. The use of pharmacotherapeutic agents to reduce pancreatic secretion is based on the concept of pancreatic feedback inhibition. There is a normal feedback loop operative in humans that controls pancreatic secretion. Although not fully elucidated, several general principles are clear and are supported by convincing experimental data. **A,** Under normal conditions, ingested protein stimulates the release of a small peptide called *cholecystokinin-releasing factor* (CCK-RF). This, in turn, stimulates the release of CCK, a potent stimulus for pancreatic enzyme secretion. CCK circulates through the blood, reaching the pancreatic acinar cells and stimulating them to secrete digestive enzymes. These enzymes reach the duodenum and begin to digest the

FIGURE 4-17.

In this study [15], normal volunteers were given a specific inhibitor of serine proteases, after which, pancreatic secretion levels were measured. Pancreatic secretion (trypsin output presented) markedly increases when an inhibitor of serine proteases is perfused in the duodenum, heat inactivating, the inhibitor returns secretion to normal. This convincingly demonstrates the presence of normal feedback, with pancreatic secretion increasing markedly when serine proteases are inhibited. (*Adapted from* Liener [15].)

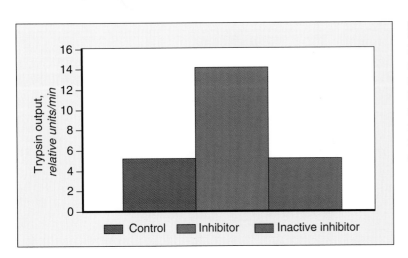

TABLE 4-4. CORRELATION OF CHOLECYSTOKININ LEVELS AND SEVERITY OF CHRONIC PANCREATITIS

	MILD TO MODERATE CHRONIC PANCREATITIS	SEVERE CHRONIC PANCREATITIS*
Fasting cholecystokinin level	↑↑	Normal or ↓
Postprandial cholecystokinin level	↑↑↑	No change or slight increase

*Marked abnormalities of main pancreatic duct (big-duct disease), diffuse calcifications, or steatorrhea.

TABLE 4-4.

Correlation of cholecystokinin (CCK) levels and severity of chronic pancreatitis. In patients with chronic pancreatitis in whom a disordered feedback is at least partially responsible for pain, elevations in CCK would be expected. Clearly, only a subset of patients with chronic pancreatitis have elevated CCK levels. Studies that have evaluated patients with more advanced disease have found normal CCK levels in many patients whereas studies evaluating patients with less advanced disease have generally demonstrated elevated levels of CCK. It is unknown why these differences occur, but it appears patients with more advanced disease have an inoperative feedback control. Whether this reflects a decrease in CCK-releasing factor, a defect in CCK production or release, or some other factor remains to be elucidated. What is clear, however, is that a substantial proportion of patients with painful chronic pancreatitis have elevated CCK levels, and it is in these patients where inhibitors of secretion are most useful.

TABLE 4-5. PANCREATIC ENZYMES AND PAIN RELIEF

CRITERIA	CONVENTIONAL	ENTERIC-COATED
Release of proteases in duodenum?	Yes	No
Lower cholecystokinin level?	Yes	No
Decrease pancreatic secretion?	Yes	No
Reduce pain?	Yes	No

TABLE 4-5.

Use of pancreatic enzymes to relieve pain. Conventional pancreatic enzymes (nonenteric-coated) are the only formulations that release their contents in the feedback-sensitive duodenum. Two randomized trials have demonstrated the efficacy of these agents for pain control [16,17]; other randomized trials using enteric-coated preparations showed no effect [18,19] surprising, inasmuch as these release their enzymes in the more distal small bowel, which is not involved in pancreatic feedback regulation. Indeed, some of these enteric-coated preparations may even stimulate pancreatic secretion! Not all patients treated with conventional enzymes responded; certain subsets appear to respond best. These subsets include patients with less-advanced disease (small-duct disease with or without absent steatorrhea), women, and patients with idiopathic chronic pancreatitis. Overall, up to 75% of carefully selected patients respond to conventional enzymes. In one study, those patients with elevated cholecystokinin (CCK) levels responded best. Although it has not yet become standard to measure CCK levels in patients with chronic pancreatitis, this may well be the most accurate way to select patients for therapy aimed at reducing secretion.

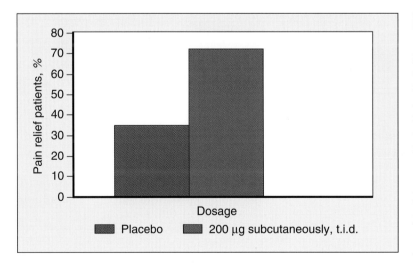

FIGURE 4-18.

Octreotide can be used to reduce pancreatic secretions and possibly relieve pain. Another method to interrupt the hyperstimulation of cholecystokinin (CCK) would be to use an inhibitor of CCK release. Octreotide, an analogue of the native hormone somatostatin, interferes with CCK release, and might be effective in reducing pain. A multicenter United States study evaluating the effect of octreotide and defining the optimum dose noted pain relief in 70% of patients on 200 µg t.i.d. subcutaneous octreotide compared with 35% of those on placebo [20]. A companion open-label study demonstrated up to 65% pain relief, with 31% of patients becoming free from pain [21]. Although still too early for general clinical use, this study has defined the appropriate dosage to be used in further studies in larger numbers of patients. A small subset of these patients had CCK levels measured. It appeared those patients who responded had elevated levels of CCK that were reduced to normal with treatment; nonresponders did not have elevated levels at baseline, and these did not change. (*Adapted from* Toskes [21].)

TABLE 4-6. PANCREATIC ENZYMES FOR THE TREATMENT OF STEATORRHEA OR PAIN

CONVENTIONAL ENZYME PREPARATIONS		ENTERIC-COATED ENZYME PREPARATIONS	
BRAND NAME	**UNITS OF LIPASE/PILL**	**BRAND NAME**	**UNITS OF LIPASE/PILL**
Lipase (Viokase)	8000	Pancrelipase (Cotazym-S)	5000
Pancrelipase (Cotazym)	8000	Enteric-coated pancrelipase (Pancrease MT4, MT10, MT16)	4000, 10,000, 16,000, respectively
Amylase (Ku-Zyme HP)	8000	Porcine pancreatic enzyme (Creon)	10,000
		Pancrelipase (Ultrase MT6, MT12, MT18, MT20)	6,000, 12,000, 18,000, 20,000, respectively

TABLE 4-6.

Enzyme use for pain. Conventional enzymes are required for the treatment of pain, but all commercially available preparations are of relatively low potency. The potency is reflected in the relative units of lipase per pill. Large numbers of pills must therefore be taken (on average, eight pills with meals and at bedtime). Because these conventional enzymes are destroyed by gastric acid, concomitant therapy with an H_2-receptor antagonist or a proton pump inhibitor is usually required. Enteric-coated preparations are the treatment of choice for steatorrhea because they are of much higher potency and do not require suppression of gastric acid.

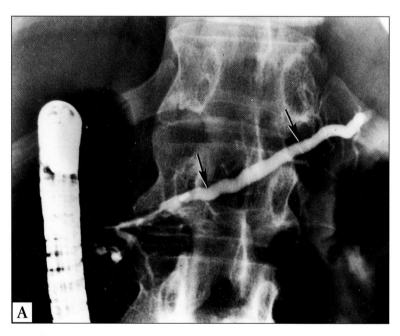

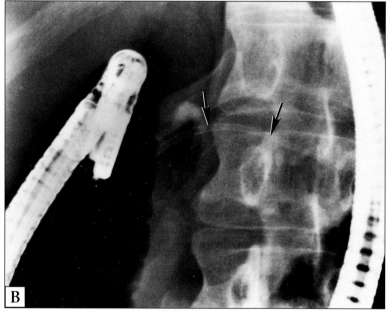

FIGURE 4-19.

Endoscopic treatment. Endoscopic treatment might include dilation of dominant strictures, removal of pancreatic ductal stones, sphincterotomy of the major or minor papilla, or pancreatic duct stenting. None of these techniques have been evaluated in a randomized trial in patients with chronic pancreatitis; in many anecdotal reports, the response rate is equivalent to the placebo response rate (approximately 35%). In addition, pancreatic duct stenting has been documented to produce chronic pancreatitis in both animal models and in humans [6,22]. Endoscopic therapy thus seems to be most amenable in patients with large obstructing pancreatic duct stones or dominant downstream strictures with upstream dilation, but the utility of endoscopic therapy in these conditions is unproven, and its use should be investigated in larger clinical trials. **A,** An injection through the minor papilla in a patient with pancreas divisum, which fills an abnormal dorsal duct (*arrows*). **B,** A stent is being placed into the dilated dorsal duct (*arrows*).

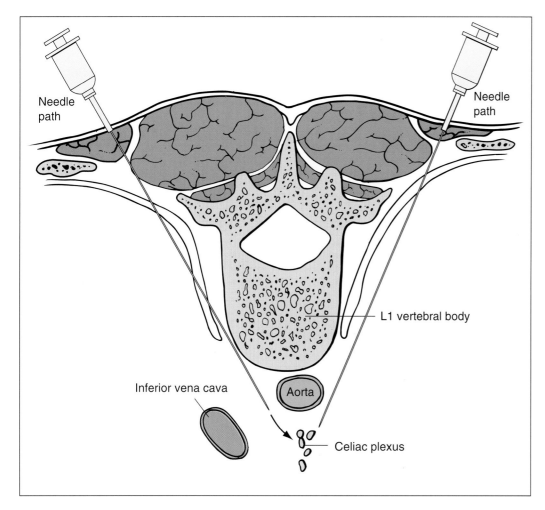

FIGURE 4-20.

Percutaneous celiac axis block for pain. Injection of the celiac nerve plexus and surgical resection of this plexus have only been evaluated in limited numbers of patients with painful chronic pancreatitis. In general, less than one third of patients respond initially and less than 10% have prolonged relief from pain. These disappointing results have produced little enthusiasm for this technique. (*Adapted from* Leung [23]; with permission.)

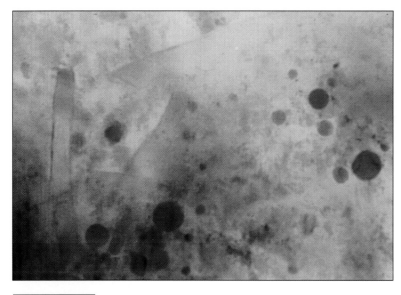

FIGURE 4-21.

Steatorrhea and diabetes. The diagnosis of steatorrhea is usually based on compatible clinical features (*eg*, diarrhea, weight loss), elimination of alternative causes (*eg*, small bowel–bacterial overgrowth), and documentation of excess fat in stool. The standard criterion is a 72-hour fecal fat collection, but this test is cumbersome and unpleasant. As a substitute, a qualitative fecal fat coupled with a response to enzyme replacement may be used to corroborate the clinical diagnosis. This figure demonstrates a stain of fecal fat, with the red-orange globules indicating the presence of excess fat. Unlike pain, steatorrhea is usually relatively easy to

manage. Enteric-coated enzymes are the treatment of choice, and two or three of the high-potency preparations with meals and snacks are usually able to improve steatorrhea. Treatments to reduce gastric acid are usually not required with enteric-coated preparations. Nutritional support may also be required in patients with significant malnutrition. Steatorrhea cannot usually be totally corrected despite the use of these enzymes, but this is not necessary to allow patients to gain weight and improve nutritional status. Use of these enzymes is safe, but there are recent reports of colonic strictures developing in patients with cystic fibrosis who were treated with the highest potency formulations in extraordinary doses. Enzyme preparations containing more than 20,000 units of lipase per pill have recently been withdrawn from the market by the manufacturers for this reason. This complication has not been reported in other patients with chronic pancreatitis.

Diabetes associated with chronic pancreatitis, particularly in patients who are chronic alcoholics, can be difficult to manage. In addition to relative insulin deficiency, these patients often continue to consume alcohol, have irregular food intake, and are often noncompliant with treatment. Treatment-associated hypoglycemia is common, and produces substantial morbidity and even mortality. Even low doses of exogenous insulin may produce hypoglycemia, perhaps because of the accompanying relative lack of glucagon. Microvascular complications, such as retinopathy, were previously believed to be uncommon, but appear in recent studies to be as common as in patients with typical diabetes mellitus if corrected for disease duration. Oral hypoglycemics are occasionally useful, but long-lasting agents should be avoided. If insulin is used, the goal should not be tight control of blood sugar, but rather the control of large urinary losses of glucose.

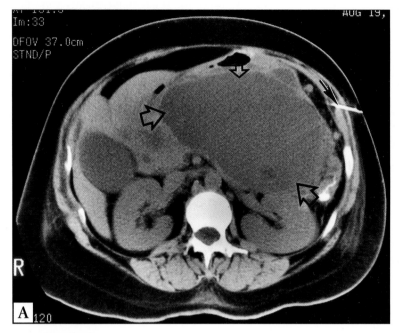 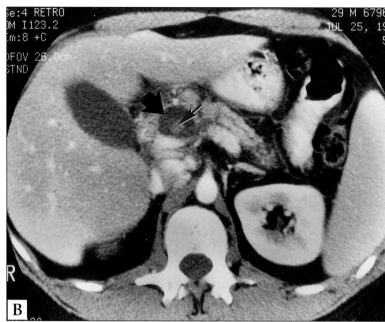

FIGURE 4-22.

Pseudocysts. **A,** A large pseudocyst (*open arrows*), which is being percutaneously drained (*closed arrow*). Pseudocysts that develop in chronic pancreatitis are most commonly caused by duct obstruction, with the formation of a "retention" cyst in the upstream duct or side branch. Unlike the pseudocysts associated with acute pancreatitis, these pseudocysts do not contain activated enzymes, and are usually not a reflection of a necrotizing inflammatory process. These pseudocysts are less likely to produce complications than those associated with acute necrotizing pancreatitis, but they are paradoxically also less likely to resolve. Many of these pseudocysts remain asymptomatic, but they may be complicated by infection, rupture or leak, bleeding, or obstruction of a neighboring hollow viscus (*eg,* duodenum, bile duct, colon, or ureter, among others). Pseudocysts may also worsen chronic pain or even initiate a wasting syndrome.

Recent clinical experience suggests that in patients with pseudocysts smaller than 6 cm, if there is a mature pseudocyst wall on radiographic imaging that does not resemble a cystic neoplasm, minimal symptoms, and no evidence of active alcohol abuse, the risk of complications is extremely small (< 10%). These patients may be safely observed with little risk of serious complication [24,25]. Even larger asymptomatic pseudocysts can be considered for expectant management in this group of patients. Symptomatic pseudocysts or those producing complications require therapy.

Surgical decompression remains the standard criterion for symptomatic pseudocysts with low mortality and little recurrence. Surgical therapy also allows the differentiation of true pseudocysts from cystic pancreatic neoplasms. Percutaneous drainage of symptomatic pseudocysts is usually successful in the short-term, but pseudocyst recurrence is common (although the recurrent pseudocyst may remain asymptomatic!). Percutaneous drainage seems to be particularly effective for infected pseudocysts; however, it is usually ineffective for other complications, such as bleeding, rupture, or leak. Bleeding is a rare event, but carries substantial mortality, often because the bleeding source is a medium-sized artery that has formed a pseudoaneurysm. **B,** A small pseudocyst in the pancreatic head (*thick arrow*) with an arterial pseudoaneurysm within it (*thin arrow*), a condition associated with the potential for massive hemorrhage. Embolization, usually followed by surgical decompression of the pseudocyst and ligation of the bleeding artery, is the treatment of choice. Rupture of a pseudocyst or the development of a leak (pancreaticopleural or other fistula) usually requires preoperative delineation of the anatomy by computed tomography or endoscopic retrograde pancreatography, followed by surgical closure and cyst enterostomy.

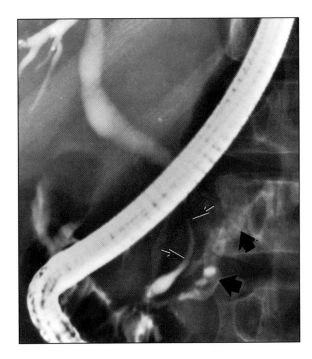

FIGURE 4-23.

Common bile duct stricture. Common bile duct stricture may develop as a consequence of compression by an adjacent pseudocyst or by progressive fibrosis of the head of the pancreas. This figure demonstrates an endoscopic retrograde cholangiopancreatography with changes of chronic pancreatitis (*thick arrows*) and a coexistent smooth stricture of the intrapancreatic common bile duct (*thin arrow*). Symptomatic obstruction of the bile duct usually requires surgical biliary bypass, usually in conjunction with a Peustow procedure.

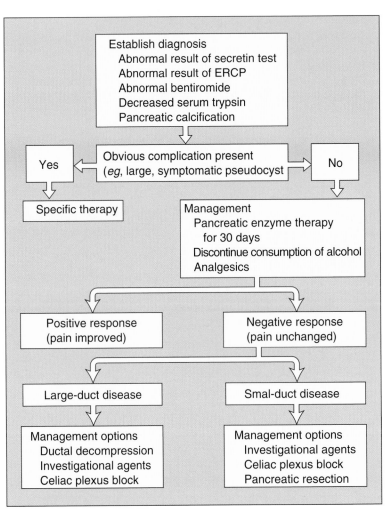

FIGURE 4-24.

Management strategy. Overall management of chronic pancreatitis requires that the diagnosis first be established. Initial evaluation should focus on defining the presence of obvious complication and in differentiating pancreatic carcinoma from chronic pancreatitis, if necessary. All patients with alcoholic chronic pancreatitis should be encouraged to stop drinking alcohol, nutritional deficiencies should be corrected, and diabetes should be treated if present. Analgesics are usually required; the least potent formulation should be tried first. A trial of conventional enzymes should usually be attempted if patients suffer from pain; although patients with advanced disease are less likely to respond to this therapy, it is without significant side-effects, and may be helpful in a subset of these patients. If medical therapy for pain is ineffective, attempts should be made to differentiate patients with small-duct disease from those with large duct disease. Patients with dilated pancreatic ducts should be considered for surgical therapy, in particular, lateral pancreaticojejunostomy. In patients who do not respond to these therapies, consideration can be given to pancreatic resection, referral to a pancreatic center, or experimental therapies (*ie*, octreotide). ERCP—endoscopic retrograde cholangiopancreatography. (*Adapted from* Forsmark and Toskes [26]; with permission.)

REFERENCES

1. Sarles H, Adler G, Dani R, *et al.*: The pancreatitis classification of Marseilles-Rome 1988. *Scand J Gastroenterol* 1989, 24:641.

2. DiMagno EP, Go VLW, Summerskill WHJ: Relationship between pancreatic enzyme output and malabsorption in severe pancreatic insufficiency. *N Engl J Med* 1973, 288:813–815.

3. Ammann RW, Akovbiantz A, Largiader F, Schueler G: Course and outcome of chronic pancreatitis: Longitudinal study of a mixed medical-surgical series of 245 patients. *Gastroenterology* 1984, 86:820–828.

4. Layer P, Yamamoto H, Kalthoff L, *et al.*: The different courses of early- and late-onset idiopathic and alcoholic chronic pancreatitis. *Gastroenterology* 1994, 107:1481–1487.

5. Axon ATR, Classen M, Cotton PB, *et al.*: Pancreatography in chronic pancreatitis: International definitions. *Gut* 1984, 25:1107–1112.

6. Forsmark CE, Toskes PP: What does an abnormal pancreatogram mean? *Gastrointest Clin North Am* 1995, 5:in press.

7. Hayakawa T, Kondo T, Shibata T, *et al.*: Relationship between pancreatic exocrine function and histologic changes in chronic pancreatitis. *Am J Gastroenterol* 1992, 87:1170–1174.

8. Walsh TN, Rode J, Theis BA, Russell RCG: Minimal change chronic pancreatitis. *Gut* 1992, 33:1566–1571.

9. Neiderau C, Grendell JH: Diagnosis of chronic pancreatitis. *Gastroenterology* 1985, 88:1973–1995.

10. Jacobson DG, Curington C, Connery K, Toskes PP: Trypsin-like immunoreactivity as a test for pancreatic insufficiency. *N Engl J Med* 1984, 310:1307–1309.

11. Copenhagen Pancreatitis Study: An interim report from a prospective epidemiological multicenter study. *Scand J Gastroenterol* 1981, 16:305–312.

12. Worning H: Incidence and prevalence of chronic pancreatitis. In *Chronic Pancreatitis*. Edited by Beger HG, Buchler M, Ditschuneit H, Malfertheiner P. Berlin-Heidelberg: Springer-Verlag; 1990:8–14.

13. Ammann RW, Buehler H, Muench R, *et al.*: Differences in the natural history of idiopathic (nonalcholic) and alcoholic chronic pancreatitis: A comparative long-term study of 287 patients. *Pancreas* 1987, 4:368–377.

14. Go VLW, Everhart JE: Pancreatitis. In *Digestive Diseases in the United States: Epidemiology and Impact*. Edited by Everhart JE. Washington, DC: U.S. Dept. of Health and Human Services; 1994:691–712.

15. Liener IE, Goodale RL, Deshmukh A, *et al.*: Effect of trypsin inhibitor from soybeans (Bowman-Birk) on the secretory activity of the human pancreas. *Gastroenterology* 1988, 94:419–427.

16. Slaff J, Jacobson D, Tillman C, *et al.*: Protease-specific suppression of pancreatic exocrine secretion. *Gastroenterology* 1984, 87:44–52.

17. Isaksson G, Ihse I: Pain reduction by an oral pancreatic enzyme preparation in chronic pancreatitis. *Dig Dis Sci* 1983, 28:97–102.

18. Halgreen H, Thorsgaard Peterson N, Worning H: Symptomatic effect of pancreatic enzyme therapy in patients with chronic pancreatitis. *Scand J Gastroenterol* 1986, 21:104–108.

19. Mossner J, Secknus R, Meyer J, *et al.*: Treatment of pain with pancreatic extracts: Results of a prospective placebo-controlled trial. *Digestion* 1992, 53:54–66.

20. Toskes PP, Forsmark CE, DeMeo MT, *et al.*: A multicenter controlled trial of octreotide for the pain of chronic pancreatitis. *Pancreas* 1993, 8:774.

21. Toskes PP, Forsmark CE, DeMeo MT, *et al.*: An open-label trial of octreotide for the pain of chronic pancreatitis. *Gastroenterology* 1994, 106:A326.

22. Gulliver DJ, Edmunds S, Baker ME, *et al.*: Stent placement for benign pancreatic diseases: Correlation between ERCP findings and clinical response. *AJR Am J Roentgenol* 1992, 159:751–755.

23. Leung JW, Bowen-Wright M, Aveling W, *et al.*: Celiac plexus block for pain, pancreatic cancer and chronic pancreatitis. *Br J Surg* 1983, 70:730–732.

24. Vitas GJ, Sarr MG: Selected management of pancreatic pseudocysts: Operative versus expectant management. *Surgery* 1992, 111:123–130.

25. Yeo CJ, Bastidas JA, Lynch-Nyhan A, *et al.*: The natural history of pancreatic pseudocysts documented by computed tomography. *Surg Gynecol Obstet* 1990, 170:411–417.

26. Forsmark CE, Toskes PP: Chronic pancreatitis. Sandoz Monograph, 1993.

Chapter 5

Surgery for Chronic Pancreatitis

STEPHEN B. VOGEL

From the surgeon's perspective, chronic pancreatitis is a fairly discrete illness with well-defined indications for surgical intervention. Over time, and in response to various stimuli, such as chronic alcohol consumption or even acute penetrating trauma, the pancreas undergoes fibrosis with or without intermittent acute inflammation eventually leading, in many cases, to partial or complete pancreatic duct obstruction. During the process, calcification of protein precipitates deposited in the pancreatic ducts leads to pancreatolithiasis. Strictures of the pancreatic duct, caused either by fibrosis or pancreatolithiasis, results in mild to moderate pancreatic duct dilatation, and eventually the "chain-of-lakes" abnormality of the main pancreatic duct. This process may take only months following pancreatic duct injury or transection, or may occur over a period of 10 to 20 years following chronic consumption of alcohol.

The clinical features, signs, and symptoms of chronic pancreatitis are directly associated with pain, physiologic pancreatic dysfunction, and the complications of chronic pancreatitis and pseudocyst formation. Years of pancreatic fibrosis with or without ductal dilatation often lead to chronic unrelenting abdominal pain, but many patients present with intermittent attacks of pain, at times with acute pancreatitis. Narcotic addiction is common. Intestinal malabsorption from pancreatic exocrine dysfunction, steatorrhea, and late adult-onset diabetes are part of the overall syndrome. Pancreatic pseudocysts occurring in 10% to 15% of patients define a secondary set of clinical signs and symptoms often necessitating surgical intervention. Most pancreatic pseudocysts perhaps develop from the evolution of the pancreatic phlegmon in necrotizing pancreatitis. A smaller but significant number of patients develop pseudocysts without evidence of recent attacks of acute pancreatitis.

From the surgeon's viewpoint, the decision to operate on patients with chronic pancreatitis is clear-cut and based on alleviation of pain, elimination of recurrent attacks of pain and pancreatitis, and specifically, treating pancreatic pseudocysts independently of complications occurring after their formation. Although many pseudocysts resolve with time, surgical lore and tradition have evolved over years of observation, especially with high-resolution computed tomography (CT) and ultrasound examination. Many patients remain relatively asymptomatic with small 2- to 3-cm pseudocysts, but in general, those cysts growing beyond 6 to 8 cm and lasting more than 6 to 8 weeks appear to have an increased incidence of complications. In past years several of these complications were catastrophic, but the evolution of percutaneous drainage methods over the last several decades has altered the natural history of pseudocysts. Despite perhaps an increasing long-term recurrence rate following percutaneous drainage, acute symptomatic, infected, or obstructing pseudocysts can be treated by percutaneous drainage, resulting in rapid resolution of the acute symptoms.

The mainstay of surgical treatment of chronic pancreatitis is internal pancreatic duct drainage in patients with moderately to widely dilated pancreatic ductal systems. In the vast majority of cases patients are symptomatic, but relatively asymptomatic patients may undergo duct drainage in an attempt to preserve pancreatic function, decrease future malabsorption, and perhaps alter the onset of insulin-dependent diabetes mellitus. These latter indications are difficult to prove, but remain relative indications for duct drainage. The standard and preferred treatment of pancreatic pseudocysts is surgical internal drainage. It is thought a majority of pseudocysts directly communicate with the main pancreatic duct, thereby leading to recurrence following either percutaneous drainage or surgical external drainage. Internal drainage leads to pseudocyst collapse, and often in the case of Roux-en-Y drainage, to ongoing decompression of pancreatic juice into the intestines.

The vast majority of patients undergoing treatment for the pain of chronic pancreatitis undergo duct drainage by longitudinal pancreatojejunostomy (Puestow's procedure). A small but significant number of patients with no evidence of duct dilatation, but with severe fibrotic chronic pancreatitis, undergo extensive pancreatic resection in the form of subtotal, or occasionally, near-total pancreatectomy with preservation of a rim of pancreas on the medial surface of the duodenum. These resective procedures are usually reserved for those patients who already suffer from insulin-dependent diabetes mellitus. In the presence of dilatation of both the pancreatic and bile ducts, and with moderate to severe inflammation at the head of the pancreas, some surgeons prefer pancreatoduodenectomy as their procedure of choice. This operation adequately decompresses both ducts in addition to offering significant pain relief. The increased morbidity of this operation relegates it in many instances to a "last procedure of choice." Pancreatoduodenectomy is the procedure of choice, however, when malignancy is suspected or cannot be ruled out, especially with no long-term history of recurrent pancreatitis. Most surgeons, however, would prefer double-duct decompression into a Roux-en-Y limb of jejunum when malignant consideration is of minimal concern.

In chronic pancreatitis there are special circumstances where diagnosis and treatment are altered by advanced imaging, early detection, and evolution of clinical experience:

Pancreatic Ascites. In the absence of acute trauma, the etiology of pancreatic ascites in most cases is caused by "leaking fluid" from a pancreatic pseudocyst. The diagnosis is confirmed following demonstration of a high amylase content in ascitic fluid. CT examination further confirms this diagnosis by demonstrating the presence of a pancreatic pseudocyst. Endoscopic retrograde cholangiopancreatography (ERCP) often demonstrates the site of leaking pancreatic fluid. Although much has been written about identification of the specific area of "leak" leading to pancreatic ascites, internal drainage of the pseudocyst results in resolution of the problem. Distal pancreatectomy is indicated for the few cases in which pancreatic ascites may be leaking from a dilated pancreatic duct. In this case, the more proximal duct is opened and internally drained into a Roux-en-Y limb of jejunum. Internal surgical drainage for a chronic pancreatic pseudocyst and pancreatic ascites is the treatment of choice. In those patients with an acute symptomatic pseudocyst or in whom the wall does not appear thick enough for internal drainage, the percutaneous approach usually results in rapid collapse of the pseudocyst and resolution of symptoms and pancreatic ascites.

Pseudoaneurysm. Hemorrhage from a visceral artery into the pseudocyst results in what is termed a *pancreatic pseudoaneurysm.* Patients often present with a history of upper gastrointestinal (GI) hemorrhage, especially if the pseudocyst communicates with the main pancreatic duct and duodenum. High-resolution imaging with the rapid delivery of intravenous dye usually demonstrates accumulations of contrast material within the pseudocyst. Initial treatment should be directed at identifying and "clotting" the visceral artery before surgical intervention. The majority of documented cases occur from either the gastroduodenal or splenic artery, but other visceral arteries, including the hepatic, right gastric, and branches of the superior mesenteric artery, can be implicated in this syndrome.

Infection. In a patient with a known pancreatic pseudocyst and clinical findings of infection, percutaneous drainage and parenteral antibiotics usually result in rapid resolution of clinical infection. In the absence of easy radiologic access to this pseudocyst, antibiotics and surgery usually address the problem. Well-defined infected pseudocysts can usually undergo internal drainage following irrigation of the cavity. Less well-defined pseudocysts with a necrotic infected wall most often undergo surgical external drainage.

Familial. Hereditary pancreatitis is now recognized in kindreds throughout the world. Extended families have been identified in Canada, Japan, and numerous areas of the United States. In most cases, CT and ERCP demonstrate massive dilatation of the main pancreatic duct, often involving the entire circumference of the gland. Huge pancreatic stones are present in the main pancreatic duct. These changes are recognized early, even in the pediatric age group, and can be adequately treated by internal surgical drainage, thus preserving pancreatic tissue and function.

Trauma. Blunt abdominal trauma often leads to partial or complete pancreatic duct disruption or transection at the midbody of the pancreas directly overlying the aorta. The early performance of a high-resolution CT examination followed by ERCP demonstrates the process. CT often demonstrates the transected midbody pancreas, but ERCP documents complete pancreatic duct transection. Early surgical intervention and pancreatic resection distal to the transection will prevent either acute symptomatic pancreatitis or the slow development of chronic pancreatitis in the distal segment.

Overall results in treating the syndrome of chronic pancreatitis are most gratifying with pain relief in approximately 70% to 85% of patients at 1 to 2 years. These results decrease over time, and most reviews have documented long-term pain relief at 50% to 60%. The problem of narcotic addiction unfortunately may specifically decrease the incidence of long-term pain relief. In the absence of drug dependency and identifying further duct dilatation by CT and ERCP, most patients with recurrent symptoms will undergo reoperation, extensive pancreatic resection, or a second attempt at duct drainage if the prior Roux-en-Y pancreatojejunostomy is no longer adequately draining the pancreatic duct. Internal surgical drainage of pancreatic pseudocysts is equally gratifying. Most surgical reviews document only a 10% to 15% recurrence rate following adequate internal decompression. Following internal drainage, upper GI examination using barium swallow demonstrates closure of pancreatic cyst gastrostomy and cyst duodenostomy anastomoses. ERCP examination following Roux-en-Y pseudocyst drainage often demonstrates continued decompression of the pancreatic gland (in the absence of proximal duct stricturing); this procedure remains our primary treatment for overall internal pseudocyst drainage.

PATHOGENESIS AND ETIOLOGY

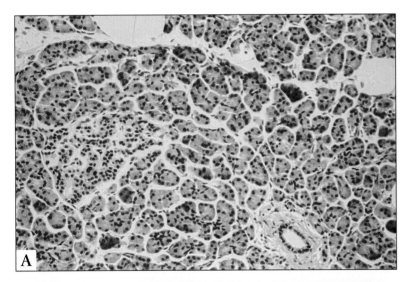

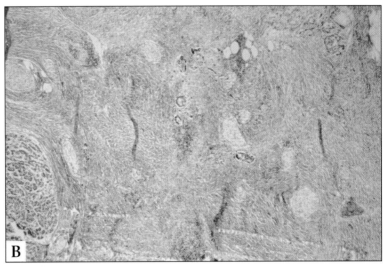

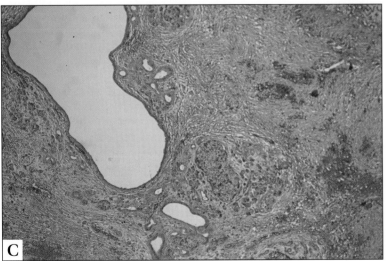

FIGURE 5-1.

A–C, Over time, and in response to various stimuli, the pancreas begins to scar, eventually undergoing moderate to severe fibrosis. The islets are the last to be affected by ongoing scar formation, yielding a significant number of patients with chronic pancreatitis who may have adult-onset, but not insulin-dependent, diabetes mellitus. This finding is important in planning a surgical approach to patients with chronic abdominal pain from chronic pancreatitis. Over a period of months to years, pancreatic ductal dilatation results from either fibrotic contraction of the gland or in response to ductal strictures with or without pancreatolithiasis. Initially, secondary or tertiary ducts begin to dilate, but eventually the main pancreatic duct undergoes moderate to severe dilatation. The chain-of-lakes ductal abnormality that is easily noted radiologically is a response to areas of ductal dilatation often separated by narrowed areas of scar or fibrosis or possibly pancreatic ductal stones partially embedded into the wall of the gland. The so-called "isthmus" between the various chains of lakes may be subtle and noted on endoscopic retrograde cholangiopancreatography only by a thinning area of contrast material. When the main pancreatic duct is opened at surgery, the importance of complete longitudinal pancreatojejunostomy becomes apparent when viewing the extremely narrowed areas of fibrosis.

TABLE 5-1. ETIOLOGY OF CHRONIC PANCREATITIS

Chronic alcohol consumption

Biliary tract disease

Blunt or penetrating trauma

Associated diseases

Early periampullary pancreatic or bile duct tumor

Familial

Idiopathic

Ampullary fibrosis

TABLE 5-1.

Alcohol consumption is the most common risk factor for developing chronic pancreatitis. Cholelithiasis, and possibly passage of stones through the ampulla, have been considered a traditional risk factor, but this concept remains speculative. Penetrating trauma (*ie*, stab wounds transecting or damaging the pancreatic duct) or blunt abdominal trauma leading to midpancreatic transection leads to the rapid development of pancreatic duct dilatation and chronic pancreatitis in some cases. Early pancreatic ductal carcinoma may present as chronic pancreatitis or recurrent attacks of acute pancreatitis. This particular group of patients often presents a preoperative and surgical dilemma. In the absence of a history of chronic alcohol ingestion, and in the presence of moderate ductal dilatation, malignancy is often suspected. A negative percutaneous or surgical biopsy does not rule out malignancy;

these patients often undergo "blind Whipple" resection when the preoperative computed tomographic (CT) or operative findings confirm resectability. I have found cancer antigen (CA) 19-9 determinations to be quite helpful in this cohort of patients. A normal or slightly elevated level does not rule out malignancy. However, CA 19-9 levels greater than 90 (in the absence of hyperbilirubinemia) confirm malignancy in over 95% of cases. Levels above 160 confirm malignancy 99% of the time. Patients with levels above 400 have either extensive or unresectable tumors regardless of preoperative CT findings. Familial or hereditary pancreatitis is a discrete illness, with findings of massive pancreatic duct dilatation and often huge pancreatic ductal stones. Following numerous attacks of acute pancreatitis, most of these patients, even in the pediatric age group, undergo internal Roux-en-Y pancreatic duct drainage. Ampullary fibrosis is perhaps a rare cause of chronic pancreatitis. Transduodenal sphincteroplasty and pancreatic ductoplasty are infrequently used in treating chronic pancreatitis. More recent radiologic imaging demonstrating ductal dilatation usually leads to duct decompression of the body and tail of the pancreas. This procedure has been used most often for postcholecystectomy syndrome and following resection of small periampullary tumors. The final category, idiopathic, is not necessarily a small and insignificant one. At least 15% of my patients undergoing blind Whipple resection for suspected pancreatic malignancy and in the presence of firmness of the entire gland have a pathologically documented severe fibrosing disease with no malignancy found in the specimen. Similarly, there is a small but significant number of patients developing chronic pancreatitis in general or pancreatic duct strictures on endoscopic retrograde cholangiopancreatography or found at surgery who have no history of alcohol consumption, biliary tract disease, or associated illnesses.

■ CLINICAL FEATURES

TABLE 5-2. SIGNS AND SYMPTOMS OF CHRONIC PANCREATITIS

Chronic abdominal and back pain

Recurrent attacks of acute pancreatitis

Pancreatic pseudocyst formation

Adult-onset diabetes

Intestinal malabsorption and steatorrhea

Abnormal liver function tests

Jaundice from bile duct obstruction

Cholangitis

TABLE 5-2.

The most common symptom of chronic pancreatitis is pain eventually developing into chronic, unrelenting abdominal pain. Many patients, however, present with intermittent attacks of abdominal pain with or without documented pancreatitis. Pain also is a predominant feature following pancreatic pseudocyst formation. Common bile duct obstruction can be caused either by fibrosis in the head of the pancreas or pseudocyst formation. The evolution of this process is usually identified by a slowly rising alkaline phosphatase determination. Endoscopic retrograde cholangiopancreatography eventually demonstrates a long narrowed stricture of the distal common bile duct. A small but significant number of patients may present with signs and symptoms of cholangitis secondary to chronic bile duct narrowing, even in the absence of clinical jaundice. In patients with recurrent attacks of right upper quadrant pain months or years following adequate internal Roux-en-Y drainage of the pancreatic duct, cholangitis and distal common bile duct narrowing should be suspected.

TABLE 5-3. RADIOLOGIC DIAGNOSIS

Computed tomography
- Pancreatic duct dilatation
- Pancreatic pseudocyst
- Degree of pancreatic inflammation

Ultrasound
- Biliary dilatation and cholelithiasis
- Pancreatic pseudocyst

Endoscopic retrograde cholangiopancreatography
- Direct evaluation of pancreatic duct and biliary system
- Demonstration of pancreatic duct strictures and chain-of-lakes formation
- Demonstrate communicating pseudocyst
- Tapered narrowing of distal common bile duct

Barium gastrointestinal examinations
- Gastrointestinal obstruction
- Pancreatic pseudocyst

TABLE 5-3.

High-resolution computed tomography (CT) and ultrasound adequately demonstrate pancreatic duct and biliary dilatation, pancreatic pseudocyst, and chain-of-lakes abnormalities. They also help delineate the tapered narrowing of the bile duct in chronic pancreatitis versus the more abrupt obstruction of malignancy. Most patients undergo ultrasound in addition to CT examination to rule out cholelithiasis. When CT adequately demonstrates pancreatic duct dilation, endoscopic retrograde cholangiopancreatography (ERCP) may be indicated to evaluate the distal common bile duct, especially in patients with an abnormal alkaline phosphatase determination. ERCP also demonstrates the degree of narrowing and dilatation in the pancreatic duct, and is helpful to the surgeon in determining the extent of the longitudinal pancreatojejunostomy procedure. In the absence of specific clinical symptoms, upper gastrointestinal examination with barium swallow is helpful in detecting early gastrointestinal narrowing or obstruction. Occasionally, pseudocysts and the chronic inflammatory process have caused obstruction in the area of the splenic flexure of the colon. In patients with a suspicious mass in the head of the pancreas, a positive result of percutaneous biopsy is significant. Negative results in biopsies are not helpful in differentiating chronic head pancreatitis versus malignancy; therefore, I usually do not recommend biopsy. Surgery is recommended for those patients with suspected malignancy, and the appropriate preoperative decision is whether resection is possible based on high-resolution CT findings.

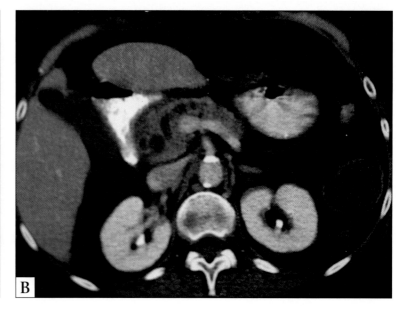

FIGURE 5-2

A–B, High-resolution spiral computed tomography with fine cuts through the pancreas adequately demonstrates pancreatic duct dilatation, even down to the ampulla, as well as demonstrating chain of lakes abnormalities.

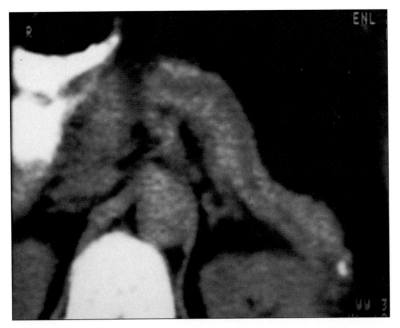

FIGURE 5-3.

Patients with chronic pancreatitis often have a small, contracted, and fibrotic pancreas. High-resolution computed tomography (CT) with fine cuts through the upper abdomen adequately demonstrates moderate pancreatic duct dilatation. If these patients are symptomatic, then these pancreatic ducts are amenable to surgical drainage and longitudinal pancreatojejunostomy. The presence of an elevated alkaline phosphatase level should suggest either preoperative endoscopic retrograde cholangiopancreatography (ERCP) to evaluate the biliary tree or intraoperative cholangiogram to perhaps demonstrate tapered stricture caused by fibrosis in the head of the pancreas. In these cases most surgeons suggest drainage of both the pancreatic and biliary systems. Although controversial, I prefer pancreatic duct drainage, even in the presence of only mild to moderate dilatation of the pancreatic duct, thereby preserving the greatest amount of pancreatic tissue and preventing conversion of adult-onset diabetes to insulin-dependent diabetes. A firm fibrotic gland with only mild to moderate duct dilatation is equally amenable to longitudinal pancreatojejunostomy and results in similar long-term results in my experience. Major resective procedures are reserved for those who remain symptomatic following the initial surgical procedure.

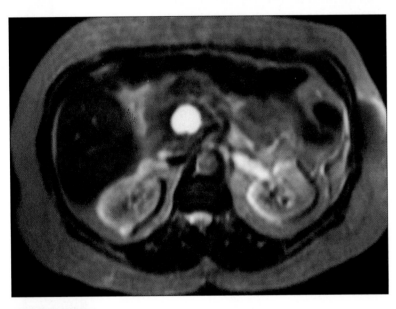

FIGURE 5-4.

Advances in MR imaging adequately demonstrate pancreatic duct abnormalities. Although these procedures are not often performed, advances in gastrointestinal and intravenous contrast material may lead to more MR imaging, especially in those patients requiring frequent computed tomographic examinations and the consideration of overall radiation dose.

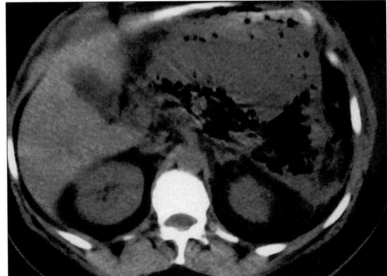

FIGURE 5-5.

Computed tomography (CT) demonstrating the "massive phlegmon" of catastrophic or necrotizing pancreatitis. This particular patient underwent surgical intervention and marsupialization of the retrogastric area. Of those patients who do not require surgical intervention, but have evidence of a massive phlegmon on CT, approximately 70% will undergo evolution to fluid collections and early pseudocyst formation. This particular group of patients with radiologic grade C or D pancreatitis on CT may comprise only 10% to 15% of all patients with pancreatitis, but may be the source of at least 80% of the total morbidity and mortality of necrotizing pancreatitis, pancreatic sepsis, and abscess formation.

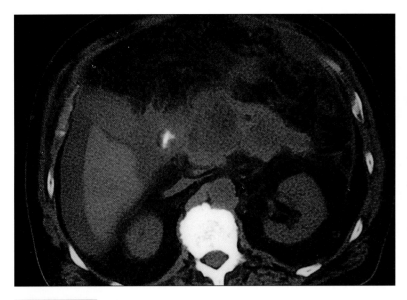

FIGURE 5-6.

Computed tomography (CT) demonstrating an evolving pancreatic phlegmon secondary to necrotizing pancreatitis in which two small pseudocysts are beginning to form. Follow-up CT in this particular patient demonstrated complete resolution of the early "pseudocyst" formation, but a larger pseudocyst may result from evolving pancreatitis of this type.

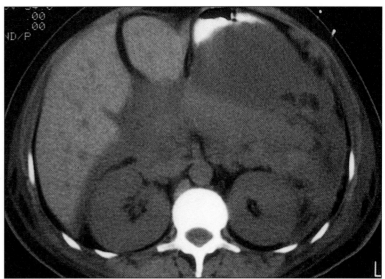

FIGURE 5-7.

Computed tomography demonstrating an acute fluid collection (or early pseudocyst formation) in evolving high-radiologic-grade pancreatitis. In those patients who are symptomatic with either pain, gastric outlet obstruction, or gastroparesis with or without persistent hypermylasemia, percutaneous drainage often results in rapid resolution of symptoms, and in most cases, normalization of the serum amylase. Continued observation of this fluid collection without intervention may demonstrate evolution of a large retrogastric pancreatic pseudocyst. Additional benefits of percutaneous drainage are the demonstration of bacteria in the fluid and recognition of early abscess formation. These particular patients usually undergo continued percutaneous drainage as long as the clinical course is improving.

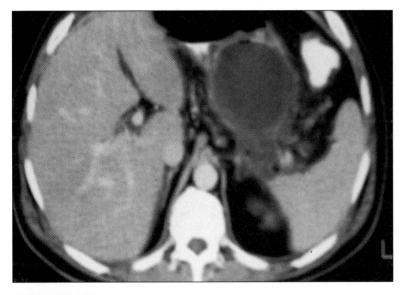

FIGURE 5-8.

High-resolution computed tomography demonstrating a chronic pancreatic pseudocyst with a thick, well-defined wall. Although percutaneous drainage may relieve the acute symptoms in this patient, long-term recurrence rates are dramatically lower following surgical internal drainage into a Roux-en-Y limb of jejunum.

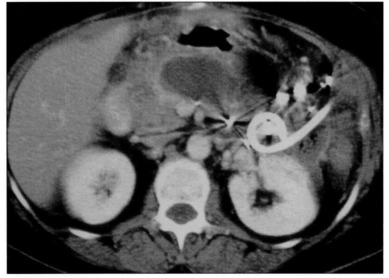

FIGURE 5-9.

Follow-up computed tomographic (CT) examination in a patient who underwent percutaneous placement of a "pig-tail" catheter into a huge flank pseudocyst. Following administration of octreotide acetate, the output rapidly diminished. Follow-up CT showed a recurrent pseudocyst in the mid-body area. Surgical internal drainage was recommended although a second (or third) catheter can be inserted to the main body of the pseudocyst following removal of the first catheter. Persistent and frequent percutaneous approaches to fluid collections may result in near complete resolution, but increase the risk of major catheter complications, including chronic infection with or without erosion into an adjacent structure. In general, surgery is recommended for recurrent pseudocyst formation.

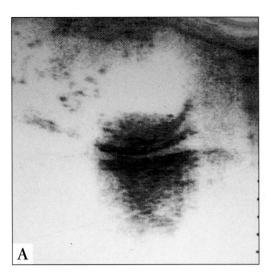 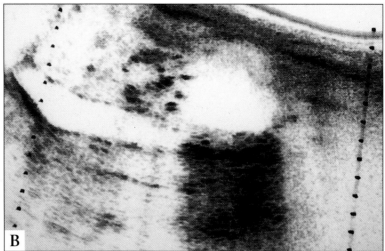

A–B, Ultrasound examination of an acutely ill patient demonstrating a pancreatic pseudocyst compressing the vena cava. The patient underwent percutaneous drainage under ultrasound guidance. Follow-up "pseudocystogram" demonstrated no communication with the main pancreatic duct, and the catheter was continued. A recurrent pseudocyst is treated surgically. If persistent percutaneous drainage results in a diminished but continued pancreatic fistula through the catheter (even following therapy with octreotide acetate), then several courses of treatment can be followed. The catheters can be removed following higher dose octreotide acetate treatment. A second surgical option is conversion of an external pancreatic fistula to internal surgical drainage. This is accomplished by changing the percutaneous catheter to a larger catheter preoperatively. This facilitates intra-abdominal identification of the fistulous tract. The tract is then "capped" as it exits the retroperitoneum and is sutured to a Roux-en-Y limb of jejunum. This technique converts the external fistula to internal drainage into the Roux-en-Y limb.

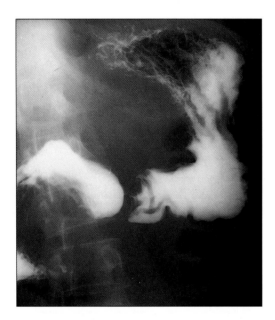

FIGURE 5-11.

Barium upper gastrointestinal (GI) examination of a patient complaining of intermittent nausea and vomiting. The patient had a previous mild attack of pancreatitis 6 months before the examination. A large pseudocyst in the head of the pancreas and pancreatic duct dilatation were demonstrated on subsequent computed tomography and endoscopic retrograde cholangiopancreatography. In this specific case the initial upper GI radiograph with barium swallow demonstrated the cause of the patient's symptoms to be an obstructing pseudocyst.

TREATMENT

TABLE 5-4. SURGERY FOR CHRONIC PANCREATITIS

Chronic pain and relapsing pancreatitis
Pancreatic pseudocysts
Biliary obstruction
Gastrointestinal obstruction
Pancreatic ascites
No specific therapy for diabetes or steatorrhea

TABLE 5-4.

Surgery is most often indicated for the long-term pain of chronic pancreatitis and its complications. The major complications include pseudocyst formation and infection, hemorrhage, or pancreatic ascites. In the absence of trauma, most patients presenting with pancreatic ascites have a pseudocyst demonstrated on computed tomography. Internal drainage of the pseudocyst results in resolution of the pancreatic ascites.

TABLE 5-5. SURGICAL PROCEDURES

Longitudinal pancreatojejunostomy (Puestow's procedure)
60%–90% pancreatic resection
Pancreatoduodenectomy ("head" pancreatitis)
Combined pancreatic duct and biliary drainage
Combined pancreatic duct and pseudocyst drainage

TABLE 5-5.

Roux-en-Y drainage of the entire pancreatic duct is the mainstay of surgical treatment. In the absence of pancreatic duct dilatation, patients can undergo a moderate to subtotal pancreatic resection. The Whipple procedure (pancreatoduodenectomy) is reserved for those few patients with inflammation in the head of the pancreas, where malignancy cannot be excluded, and who appear surgically resectable. In the presence of easily entered pseudocysts and where the pancreatic duct can also be identified, Roux-en-Y drainage of

both the pseudocyst and duct is appropriate. In most cases, however, the surgeon may encounter only the large pancreatic pseudocyst even though the communication between the duct and pseudocyst was easily demonstrated on endoscopic retrograde cholangiopancreatography (ERCP). For those patients with abnormal liver function tests and a long, tapered stricture of the bile duct on ERCP, combined pancreatic duct and biliary drainage into the same Roux-en-Y limb is the procedure of choice. As previously described, major resective procedures (60%–90% pancreatic resection) are reserved for those patients with no demonstrable pancreatic duct dilatation and usually a firm contracted fibrotic gland. Pancreatoduodenectomy for the pain of "head pancreatitis" adequately decompresses both pancreatic and bile ducts, but is less frequently performed by most surgeons, who usually prefer double-duct decompression into a Roux-en-Y limb. In selected cases most of the head of the pancreas can be resected with preservation of a rim of pancreas and the duodenum. The distal pancreas undergoes drainage into a Roux-en-Y limb. This procedure removes the source of chronic abdominal pain and preserves the duodenum and the distal pancreas, but in the presence of extensive inflammation, may lead to increased morbidity and is infrequently performed.

TABLE 5-6. PANCREATIC PSEUDOCYSTS

Roux-en-Y cystojejunostomy (internal drainage)
Cystogastrostomy
Cystoduodenostomy
Distal pancreatectomy (cyst in tail)
Percutaneous drainage for acute symptomatic pseudocysts

TABLE 5-6.

Most patients with chronic pseudocysts beyond 6 to 8 weeks of duration and above 6 to 8 cm in size usually undergo elective surgical internal drainage. The procedure of choice is Roux-en-Y drainage of any pseudocyst that can be easily reached by the Roux-en-Y limb of intestine. The cystogastrostomy procedure should be performed only when the pseudocyst is densely adherent to the posterior wall of the stomach and when Roux-en-Y drainage is difficult. The cystogastrostomy anastomosis closes rapidly in the postoperative period, although it is an adequate procedure for pseudocyst decompression. Endoscopic retrograde cholangiopancreatography (ERCP) data suggest that in the presence of a communicating pseudocyst the Roux-en-Y cystojejunostomy should remain open long term. Cystoduodenostomy can be performed for pancreatic pseudocysts in the head of the pancreas. This procedure, however, necessitates opening the medial wall of the duodenum, and may place the distal common bile duct with or without gastro-

duodenal artery in jeopardy. For this reason, Roux-en-Y drainage is preferred. Distal pancreatectomy (usually with splenectomy) is performed for pseudocysts in the tail of the pancreas. If preoperative ERCP demonstrates no proximal obstruction, then the body or tail of the pancreas may be closed. If proximal stricutres *are* demonstrated, distal pancreatectomy is combined with a more proximal longitudinal pancreatojejunostomy for adequate duct decompression. Percutaneous drainage of acute or subacute symptomatic pseudocysts results in rapid resolution of symptoms and early discharge from the hospital. The actual recurrence rate may be as high as 40% to 50%, but the ensuing chronic pseudocyst can then be surgically drained electively. Percutaneous drainage of fluid collections in acutely symptomatic patients is preferred over the standard treatment of parenteral hyperalimentation over a prolonged period to allow the pseudocyst to "mature." If the patient is well enough to be discharged home, then this form of treatment is preferred. If, however, the patient requires hospitalization, then percutaneous drainage expedites the care of the patient and facilitates early discharge from the hospital. In most cases, the percutaneous catheters are discontinued, especially with a decrease in daily volume following octreotide acetate therapy. Follow-up ultrasound and CT examinations are scheduled. Recurrent, small-fluid collections in asymptomatic patients are followed with repeat ultrasound examinations. The treatment of large, recurrent fluid collections is usually surgical with internal Roux-en-Y drainage planned. Overall recurrence of pancreatic pseudocysts following surgical internal drainage is less than 10% to 15%. These data have remained relatively constant for the past 30 years.

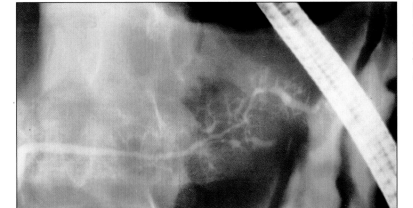

FIGURE 5-12.

Endoscopic retrograde cholangiopancreatography demonstrating a normal caliber duct with evidence of chronic changes in the tail with a small cystic formation. This patient underwent distal pancreatectomy and splenectomy with excellent relief of symptoms.

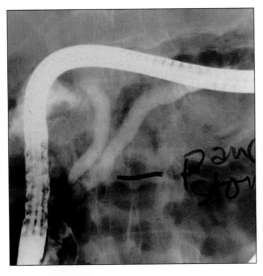

FIGURE 5-13.

Endoscopic retrograde cholangiopancreatography (ERCP) demonstrating
moderate pancreatic duct dilatation and
a suggestion of pancreatolithiasis near
the duodenum. Preoperative endoscopy
(combined with ERCP) must rule out periampullary tumors. This particular case
represents the surgical dilemma, especially
if a small mass is palpated in the head of
the pancreas or ampullary area. In cases
such as this, a pancreatoduodenectomy
may be performed when the suspicion of
early malignancy cannot be eliminated.
Malignancy should be suspected even in
patients with a recent history consistent
with chronic pancreatitis.

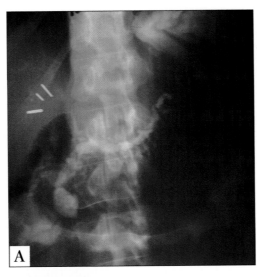
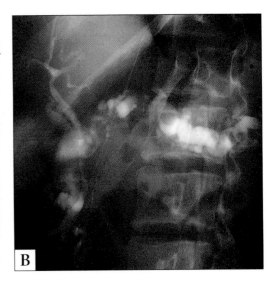

FIGURE 5-14.

Endoscopic retrograde cholangiopancreatography (ERCP) demonstrating moderate to
severe pancreatic duct abnormalities in patients with chronic pancreatitis. The "thin
contrast areas" seen in **panel A** represent stricturing of the pancreatic duct, and were
confirmed at surgery. The patient in **panel B** has a massive chain-of-lakes abnormality in
the hugely dilated distal pancreatic duct. Large pancreatic stones were demonstrated at
surgery, and retrospectively were identified on ERCP in the mid-pancreas area. Both
patients underwent longitudinal pancreatojejunostomy. The ERCP view in **panel B**
demonstrated no abnormalities in the biliary ductal system. There is a suggestion of a
large pancreatic stone in this patient, who had a history of hereditary pancreatitis.

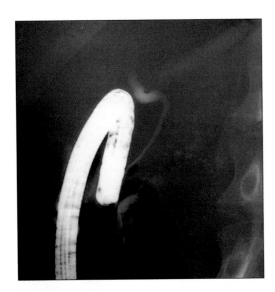

FIGURE 5-15.

Endoscopic retrograde cholangiopancreatography (ERCP) in a patient with a known
pseudocyst in the head of the pancreas. The
tapering of the distal common bile duct may
result from either the pseudocyst or from
fibrosis in the head of the gland. The pseudocyst does not communicate with the proximal

pancreatic duct, but the proximal duct is
completely strictured. Computed tomography
demonstrated a dilated distal pancreatic duct.
Surgical options include either pseudocyst
drainage alone or pseudocyst drainage
combined with longitudinal pancreatojejunostomy and possibly biliary decompression. At surgery an intraoperative cholangiogram can be performed following
pseudocyst decompression to evaluate the
distal common bile duct. If the long tapered
narrowing is persistent, then simultaneous
biliary decompression is indicated. If the
common bile duct appears normal following
pseudocyst decompression, then either
pseudocyst drainage only or pseudocyst
drainage combined with a Puestow procedure
can be performed (*see* Fig. 5-24). In selected
cases an intraoperative "pseudocystogram"
can be performed to evaluate whether
pseudocyst drainage alone will also decom-
press the distal dilated pancreatic duct. If no
communication is demonstrated between the
pseudocyst and the pancreatic duct, then an
attempt should be made to drain the distal
pancreatic duct independently.

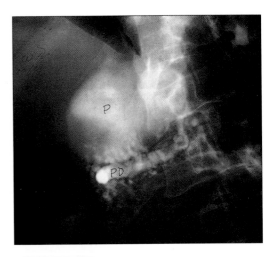

FIGURE 5-16.

Endoscopic retrograde cholangiopancreatography (ERCP) demonstrating a dilated
pancreatic duct and a huge pseudocyst in the
area of the body of the pancreas. At surgery
only the pseudocyst could easily be identified and drained. The preoperative ERCP,
however, suggested that drainage of the
pseudocyst into a Roux-en-Y would continue
to drain the body and tail of the pancreas.

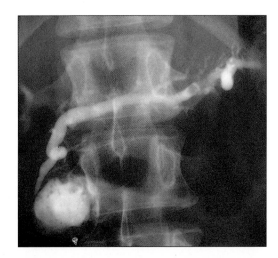

FIGURE 5-17.

Endoscopic retrograde cholangiopancreatography (ERCP) demonstrating a dilated pancreatic duct in a patient with chronic pancreatitis and a small pseudocyst in the head and uncinate process of the pancreas, communicating with the main pancreatic duct. Longitudinal pancreatojejunostomy adequately decompressed the small pseudocyst.

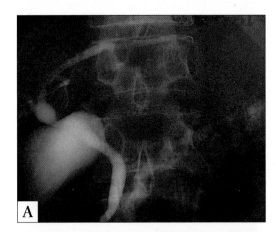

A

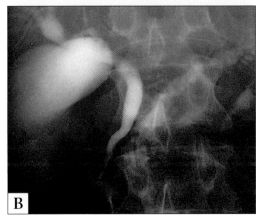

B

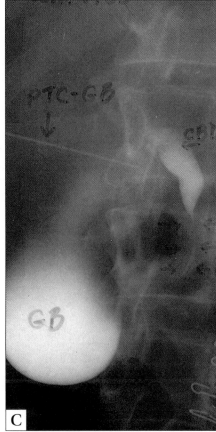

C

FIGURE 5-18.

A–C, Endoscopic retrograde cholangiopancreatography (ERCP) demonstrating changes of chronic pancreatitis and dilatation of the main pancreatic duct. Over time, fibrosis in the head of the pancreas resulted in tapering of the distal common bile duct, and biliary dilatation was demonstrated on a second ERCP 1 year following the initial examination. This patient underwent a combined longitudinal pancreatojejunostomy and biliary decompression using gallbladder anastomosis to the same Roux-en-Y limb.

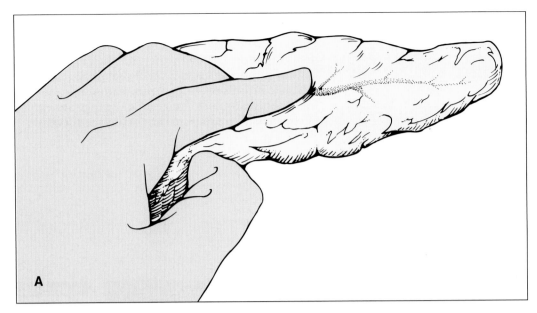

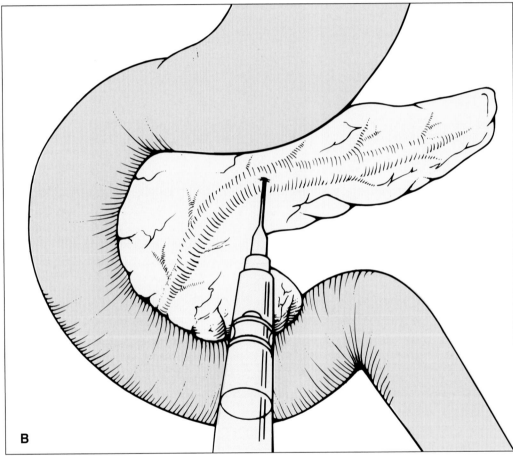

At the time of surgery most dilated pancreatic ducts can be palpated along the anterior
surface of the pancreas (**panel A**). A small syringe and needle are used to aspirate different
areas on the surface of the pancreas selectively until a small amount of pancreatic juice
enters the hub of the needle (**panel B**).

(*continued on next page*)

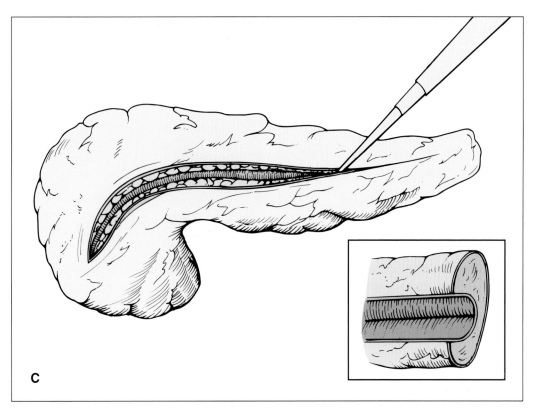

C

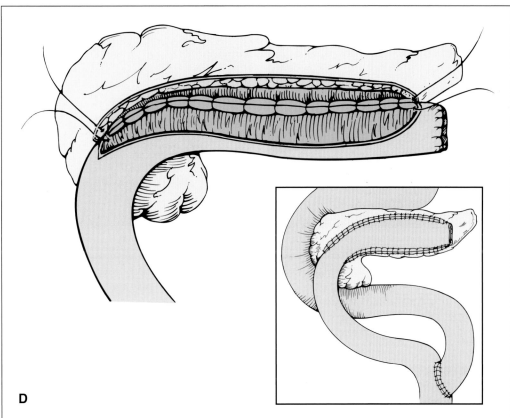

D

FIGURE 5-19. (CONTINUED)

Using electrocautery, an incision is made into the pancreas beside the needle until the pancreatic duct is entered (**panel C**). The pancreatic duct is opened in both directions. This procedure is performed to an intact pancreas or following distal pancreatectomy. A Roux-en-Y limb of jejunum is placed either to the open end of the resected pancreas or in a longitudinal fashion sutured to and covering the entire pancreatic duct (**panel D**). In most cases the pancreas is firm and fibrotic; a single-layer anastomosis is performed to the pancreatic wall, which often includes a portion of the pancreatic duct.

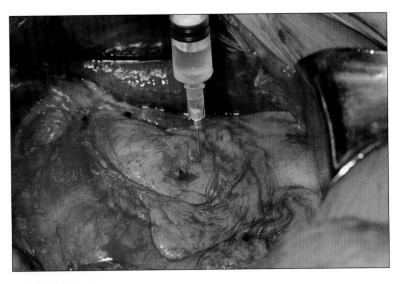

FIGURE 5-20.

The anterior surface of the pancreatic area is palpated with identification of the possible pancreatic duct. This is confirmed by aspiration of fluid.

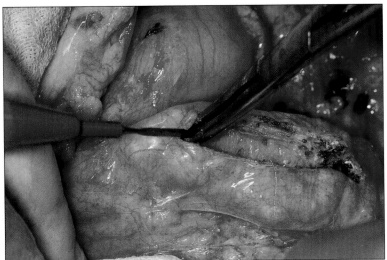

FIGURE 5-21.

After entering the pancreatic duct, electrocautery is used to open the duct in a longitudinal fashion to within 1 to 2 cm of the duodenal wall.

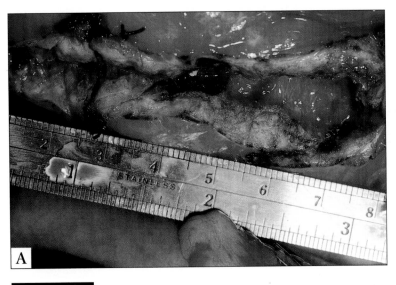

A

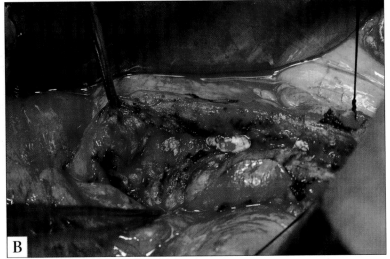

B

FIGURE 5-22.

A–B, The fibrosis and calcification of chronic pancreatitis produce numerous areas of stricture caused either by the scarring or occasionally by calcified pancreatic stones. For this reason the entire pancreatic duct is opened from the tail to approximately 1 cm from the duodenum, where the pancreatic duct curves downward

toward the ampulla of Vater. The relative obstruction shown in **panel B** would result in less than satisfactory results if distal pancreatic drainage alone was performed. In this case, the etiology of obstruction was pancreatic stones embedded in the fibrotic strictures.

FIGURE 5-23.

The longitudinal incision over the pancreatic duct is carried onto the head of the pancreas, exposing a pseudocyst involving the head and uncinate process. Both the pancreatic duct and pseudocyst are drained into a Roux-en-Y limb.

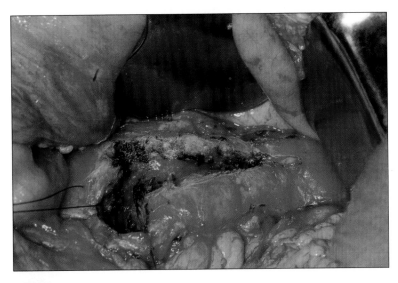

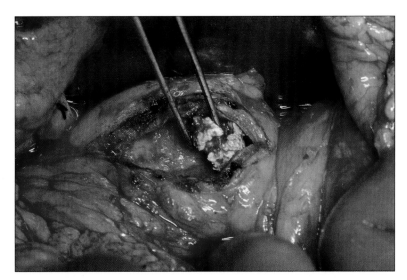

FIGURE 5-24.

A massively dilated pancreatic duct in a patient with hereditary pancreatitis demonstrating huge pancreatic stones forming within the duct and occasionally embedded in the wall of the pancreas. Longitudinal pancreatojejunostomy in this patient resulted in complete resolution of the symptoms of both chronic and acute relapsing pancreatitis.

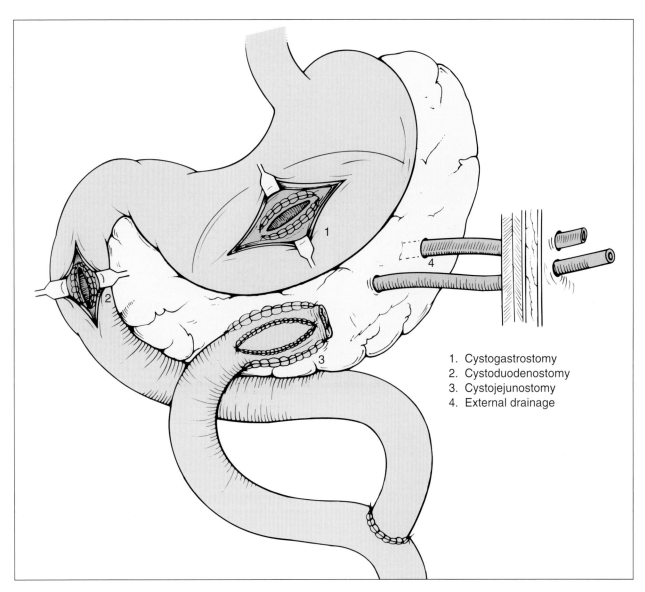

1. Cystogastrostomy
2. Cystoduodenostomy
3. Cystojejunostomy
4. External drainage

FIGURE 5-25.

The four types of procedures used to drain pancreatic pseudocysts surgically are demonstrated. Roux-en-Y internal drainage is preferred. The cystogastrostomy procedure is performed following opening into the pseudocyst through the posterior wall of the stomach and resecting an ellipse of tissue. This procedure is performed only when the pancreatic pseudocyst adheres to the back wall of the stomach. External surgical drainage has been performed when the wall of the pseudocyst is found to be too flimsy to tolerate suturing adequately. This procedure results in similar statistics, as are now being accumulated for percutaneous drainage. In the past this was the preferred treatment for pseudocysts found to be either infected or grossly necrotic. Surgical drainage into either a Roux-en-Y limb of intestine or the stomach has similar low recurrence rates of only 10% to 15%.

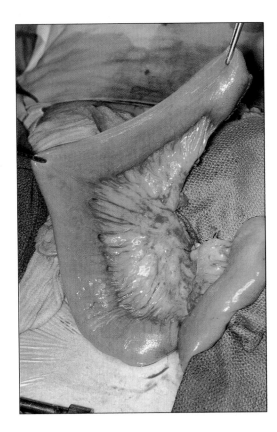

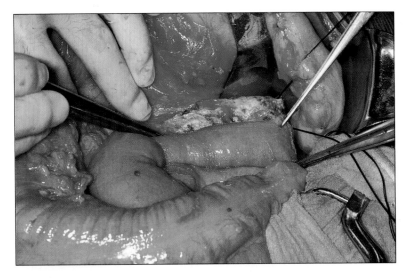

FIGURE 5-26.

The Roux-en-Y limb can be used to drain internally either the pancreatic duct alone or in combination with either the pseudocyst alone or combined with the biliary system.

FIGURE 5-27.

This patient underwent a distal pancreatectomy with proximal longitudinal pancreatojejunostomy. Preoperative endoscopic retrograde cholangiopancreatography demonstrated a moderately dilated common bile duct; the patient's alkaline phosphatase level was over 400. Following pancreatojejunostomy, the downstream portion of jejunum was anastomosed to the gallbladder as a form of biliary enteric anastomosis.

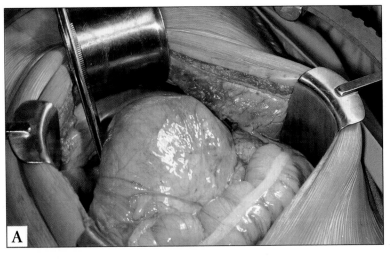

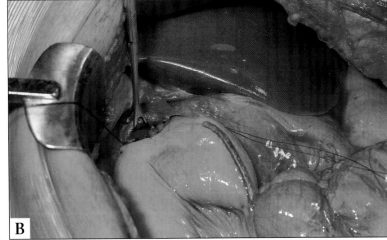

FIGURE 5-28.

A–B, This patient presented with chronic abdominal pain, evidence of partial gastric outlet obstruction, and an elevated alkaline phosphatase level. In the history there were several episodes of right upper quadrant pain, chills, and fever. Ultrasound demonstrated a dilated common bile duct and gallbladder, and computed tomographic examination demonstrated a huge pancreatic pseudocyst encompassing the narrowed duodenum in the right upper quadrant surrounding a narrowed duodenum. Following internal drainage into a Roux-en-Y limb, the patient's symptoms resolved, liver functions normalized, and follow-up ultrasound demonstrated a normal-caliber bile duct. The patient was discharged, tolerating a regular diet with no evidence of gastric outlet obstruction.

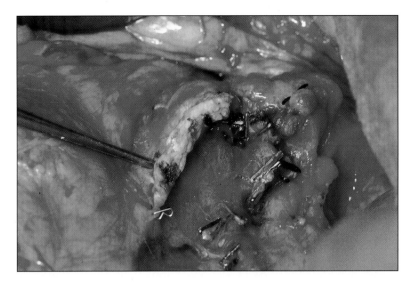

FIGURE 5-29.

Computed tomography examination demonstrated a small, sunken, fibrotic pancreas in this patient with a long history of alcohol consumption and chronic unrelenting abdominal pain. Endoscopic retrograde cholangiopancreatography demonstrated a narrow but abnormal pancreatic duct. The patient underwent subtotal pancreatectomy to include the body and tail and a portion of the head of the pancreas to the right of the visualized portal vein. Most of the fibrotic uncinate process and a small limb of pancreas were spared. This figure demonstrates the narrowed, fibrotic pancreas as it was dissected from the portal vein.

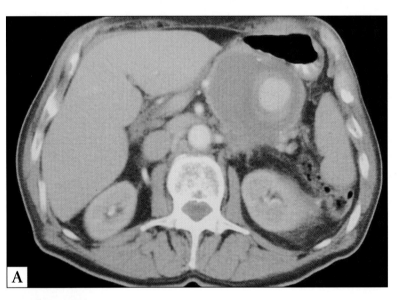

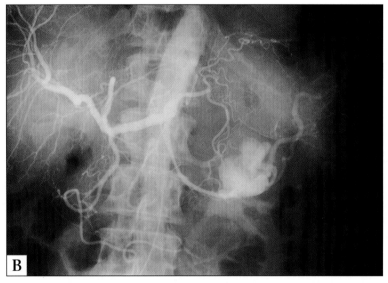

FIGURE 5-30.

A, Computed tomographic view in a patient with a history of prior pancreatitis, present left upper-quadrant pain, and anemia. Intravenous contrast is demonstrated in a large pancreatic pseudocyst. B, Preoperative arteriogram demonstrates "leaking" contrast material from the splenic artery into the pseudocyst. The splenic artery was preoperatively "clotted" using a combination of metal coils and Gelfoam. The patient underwent Roux-en-Y internal drainage of a pseudocyst. Findings at surgery confirmed the presence of old clot formation with evidence of recent hemorrhage.

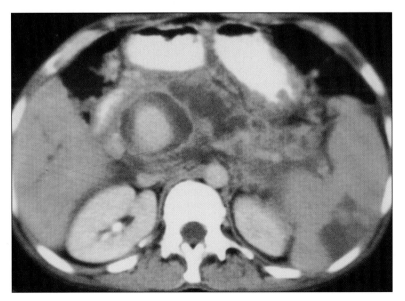

FIGURE 5-31.

This patient presented with a history of recent upper gastrointestinal hemorrhage and a history of long-term heavy alcohol consumption. Computed tomography demonstrated accumulation of dye in the head of the pancreas; angiography documented a pseudoaneurysm of the pseudocyst originating from the gastroduodenal artery. Before surgery, the gastroduodenal artery was clotted with metal coils placed superiorly and inferiorly surrounding the area of extravasation. Subsequently, the patient underwent surgical Roux-en-Y internal drainage.

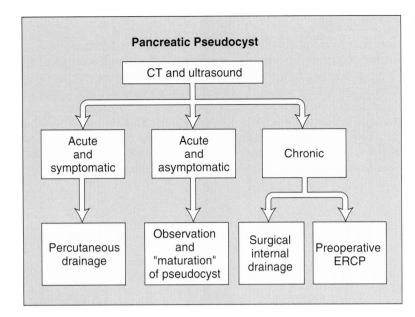

Pancreatic Pseudocyst

CT and ultrasound

Acute and symptomatic → Percutaneous drainage

Acute and asymptomatic → Observation and "maturation" of pseudocyst

Chronic → Surgical internal drainage / Preoperative ERCP

FIGURE 5-32.

Most patients with pancreatic disease in general, or pancreatic pseudocyst specifically, will undergo one or more computed tomography (CT) and ultrasound examinations during the course of their disease. In these patients with acute, symptomatic early pseudocyst formation (or fluid collections) who cannot be discharged from the hospital, percutaneous drainage is the preferred initial treatment as the most expeditious means of resolving the patient's symptoms and facilitating early discharge. In those patients with acute pseudocyst formation who are relatively asymptomatic and can be discharged from the hospital, nonsurgical treatment with follow-up CT or ultrasound examination is recommended. Many of these pseudocysts will resolve over time so long as the patient remains asymptomatic. Although many early pseudocysts have an adequate wall for surgical internal drainage, conservative observations may result in complete resolution of the process. When chronic pseudocysts persist, surgical internal drainage is recommended, although as previously described, percutaneous drainage can be performed for numerous pseudocyst complications or even for pseudocysts without complications with some degree of success in long-term follow-up. ERCP—endoscopic retrograde cholangiopancreatography.

TABLE 5-7. CHRONIC PANCREATITIS

Total pancreatobiliary drainage

Preservation of pancreatic function delays insulin dependence

Avoids major resective procedures

Combined drainage of pseudocyst bile duct and dilated pancreatic duct

TABLE 5-7.

Although numerous procedures have been described for the treatment of chronic unrelapsing abdominal pain in patients with chronic pancreatitis, my preferred treatment as described is total pancreatobiliary drainage in the appropriate patient. The main thrust of this approach is preservation of as much pancreatic tissue as possible during the primary surgical procedure. We feel that this approach avoids major resective procedures, delays the onset of insulin-dependent diabetes, may delay the onset of steatorrhea (although this remains speculative), and can be safely performed. In most cases the same Roux-en-Y limb that is used in performing the procedure of longitudinal pancreatojejunostomy can also drain noncommunicating pseudocysts and dilated bile ducts caused by fibrosis in the head of the pancreas. We have also performed these procedures not only for major pancreatic duct dilatation, but in most cases of mild to moderate dilatation. As described, major resective procedures are reserved for those patients with no ductal dilatation, a small fibrotic and contracted pancreas, or in cases where malignancy cannot be excluded. Because of the firm nature of pancreatic tissue, pancreatic leaks following anastomosis are rare and longitudinal pancreatojejunostomy can be performed safely with minimal morbidity. Overall pseudocyst recurrence rates following internal drainage represent only 10% to 15% of patients in a long-term follow-up. Overall pain relief following longitudinal pancreatojejunostomy for chronic pancreatitis alone is quite reasonable, with early successful results of 75% to 85%.

▮ SELECTED BIBLIOGRAPHY

Adler J, Barkin JS: Management of pseudocysts, inflammatory masses, and pancreatic ascites. *Gastroenterol Clin North Am* 1990, 19:863–871.

Ammann RW, Buehler H, Muench R, *et al.*:Differences in the natural history of idiopathic (nonalcoholic) and alcoholic chronic pancreatitis: A comparative long-term study of 287 patients. *Pancreas* 1987, 2:368–377.

Becker JM: Pancreatic pseudocyst. In *Current Surgical Therapy*, edn. 4. Edited by Cameron JL. St. Louis: Mosby-Year Book; 1992:423–426.

Bradley EL: Pancreatic cystenterostomy. In *Master of Surgery*, edn 3. Edited by Nyhus LM, Baker RJ, Fischer JE. Boston: Little Brown; 1997:1224–1232.

Greenlee HB, Prinz RA, Aranha GV: Long-term results of side-to-side pancreaticojejunostomy. *World J Surg* 1990, 14:70–76.

Nealon WH, Townsend CM, Thompson JC: Preoperative endoscopic pancreatic pseudocyst associated with resolving acute and chronic pancreatitis. *Ann Surg* 1989, 209:532–538.

Prinz RA, Deziel DJ: Roux en Y lateral pancreaticojejunostomy for chronic pancreatitis. In *Master of Surgery*, edn 3. Edited by Nyhus LM, Baker RJ, Fischer JE. Boston: Little Brown; 1997:1205–1214.

Rossi RL, Schirmer WJ: Chronic pancreatitis. In *Current Surgical Therapy*, edn. 4. Edited by Cameron JL. St. Louis: Mosby-Year Book; 1992:431–441.

Van Sonnenberg E, Wittich GR, Casola G, *et al.*: Percutaneous drainage of infected and non-infected pancreatic pseudocysts: Experience in 101 cases. *Radiology* 1980, 170:757–761.

Yeo CJ, Bastidas JA, Lynch-Nyhan A, *et al.*: The natural history of pancreatic pseudocysts documented by computed tomography. *Surg Gynecol Obstet* 1990, 170:411–417.

Chapter 6

Developmental Anomalies of the Pancreas

GLEN A. LEHMAN

Developmental anomalies are, by definition, present at birth but commonly are not suspected or detected until adulthood. The term *developmental anomaly* indicates that during embryologic maturation there was atypical development, and in the final analysis, an abnormality occurred, which by implication may cause some disease, limitation, or disability. Congenital alterations that are generally of limited clinical importance might best be termed *congenital variations*. In reality, most developmental anomalies and variants of the pancreas are of no clinical significance and are detected coincidentally at endoscopy, surgery, or autopsy. In selected settings, these alterations have clinical consequences and are the focus of this chapter. This chapter focuses mostly on adult patients. Although significant congenital anomalies of the pancreas presenting in childhood are generally detected by computed tomographic scans, barium studies, or laparotomy, endoscopic detection and management are being increasingly used [1–4].

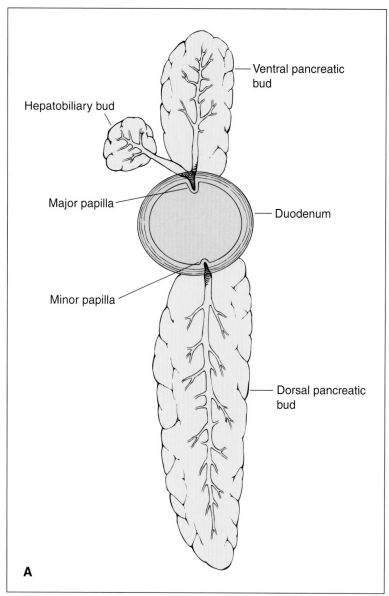

Ventral pancreatic bud

Hepatobiliary bud

Major papilla

Duodenum

Minor papilla

Dorsal pancreatic bud

A

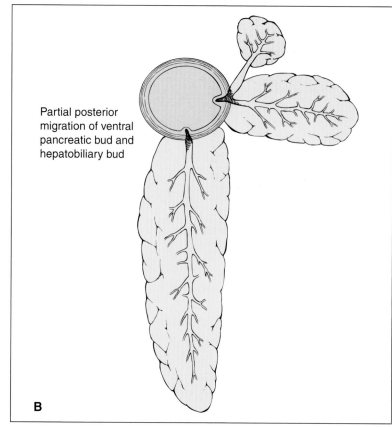

Partial posterior migration of ventral pancreatic bud and hepatobiliary bud

B

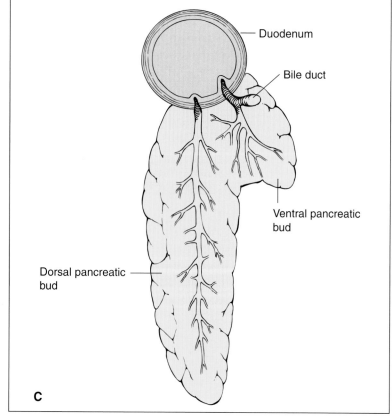

Duodenum

Bile duct

Ventral pancreatic bud

Dorsal pancreatic bud

C

FIGURE 6-1.

A, Embryologic development of the ventral and dorsal pancreas as it occurs in the fourth to eighth weeks of intrauterine development. **B,** The ventral bud gives rise to the hepatobiliary tree and the ventral pancreas, whereas the dorsal bud gives rise only to the dorsal pancreas. **C,** The ventral pancreas rotates posteriorly to the duodenum and comes to lie posteriorly and inferiorly to the dorsal pancreas. Parenchymal fusion of the two pancreatic buds nearly always occurs, but ductal nonfusion is more common, although it has not yet occurred in this view.

(*continued on next page*)

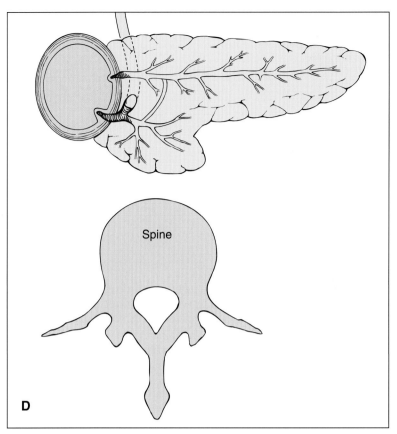

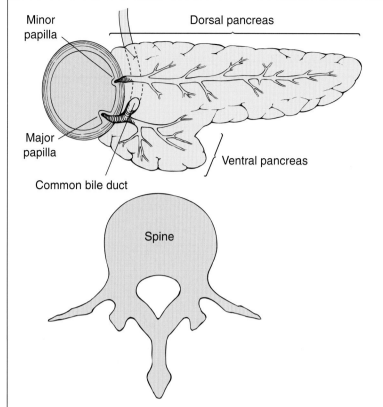

FIGURE 6-1. (CONTINUED)

D, Duodenal rotation has occurred, as well as pancreatic dorsal and ventral ductal fusion. Structures lie in their normal adult position, as would be seen on computed tomographic scan [5].

FIGURE 6-2.

Diagrammatic view of pancreas divisum, as seen in computed tomography. The parenchyma of the ventral and dorsal pancreas are fused, but the ductal system remains separated.

TABLE 6-1.

Full classification of developmental anomalies of the pancreas.

TABLE 6-1. ANATOMIC CATEGORIZATION OF CONGENITAL PANCREATIC ANOMALIES AND VARIANTS

Ventral-dorsal ductal malfusion
  Pancreas divisum
  Incomplete pancreas divisum
  Isolated dorsal segment
Rotation-migration problems
  Annular pancreas
  Ectopic pancreas
  Ectopic papillae
Quantitative underdevelopment
  Agenesis
  Hypoplasia
Duplication
  Ductal
    Total
    Partial—tail, body
  Accessory papilla

Atypical ductal configuration
  Ansa
  Spiral
  Horseshoe
  Miscellaneous
Anomalous pancreatobiliary junction
Cystic malformations
  Single
  Polycystic

TABLE 6-2. PANCREAS DIVISUM

Occurs in 7% of whites

Occurs in 1%–2% of blacks and Asians

Results from malunion of dorsal and ventral ductal systems in utero

Alternatively called the dominant dorsal ductal system

Of pancreas divisum patients, 15% have incomplete divisum

TABLE 6-2.

Pancreas divisum.

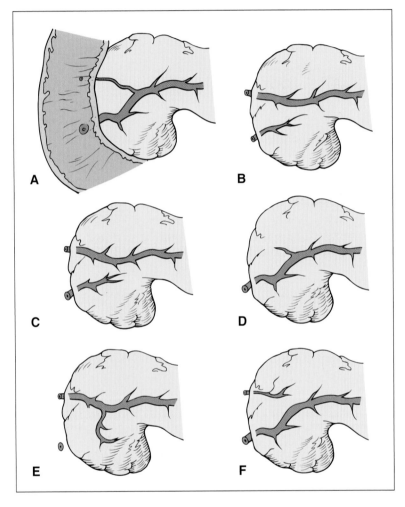

FIGURE 6-3.

Variations of pancreatic ductal anatomy, including pancreas divisum. **A**, Most common variant with patent main and accessory ducts and patent major and minor papillae. **B**, Typical pancreas divisum. **C**, Incomplete pancreas divisum. A tiny branch connects the dorsal and ventral portions of the pancreas. **D**, Minor papilla is not patent. **E**, The entire ductal system drains through the minor papilla. **F**, Isolated accessory duct system draining through the minor papilla.

TABLE 6-3. CLINICAL SIGNIFICANCE OF PANCREAS DIVISUM

TABLE 6-3.

Clinical significance of pancreas divisum [8–13].

Only ventral ductal system is seen through major papilla ductography

Ventral pancreatogram must be differentiated from obstructed duct of cancerous or benign stricture

In select cases, the minor papilla orifice is critically small and obstructs the flow of exocrine juice, causing pain or pancreatitis

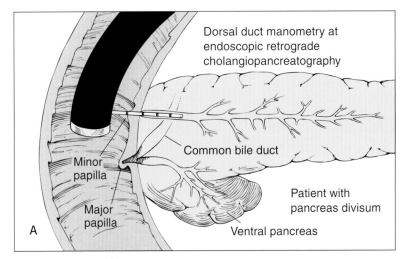

Dorsal duct manometry at endoscopic retrograde cholangiopancreatography

Common bile duct

Minor papilla

Major papilla

Patient with pancreas divisum

Ventral pancreas

A

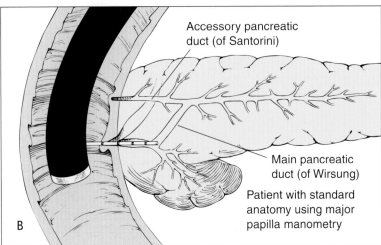

Accessory pancreatic duct (of Santorini)

Main pancreatic duct (of Wirsung)

Patient with standard anatomy using major papilla manometry

B

FIGURE 6-4.

Staritz has measured intraductal pressure through the minor and major papillae and has shown that intraductal pressure (dorsal duct) in patients with pancreas divisum (**panel A**) is approximately twice as high as intraductal pressures measured in patients who do not have pancreas divisum (**panel B**) [14].

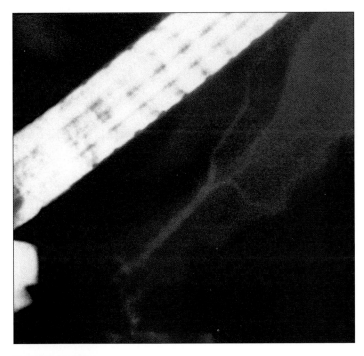

FIGURE 6-5.

Typical ventral ductogram of pancreas divisum showing small ductal system, which terminates in small-caliber branches.

FIGURE 6-6.

Another small, normal ventral ductogram. Slight acinarization has occurred.

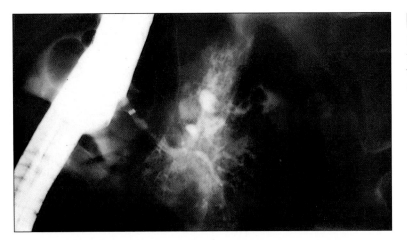

FIGURE 6-7.

Pancreatic cancer involving the head of the gland, which obstructs the duct and produces a short ductogram somewhat similar to the ventral duct seen in pancreas divisum. Acinarization has also occurred.

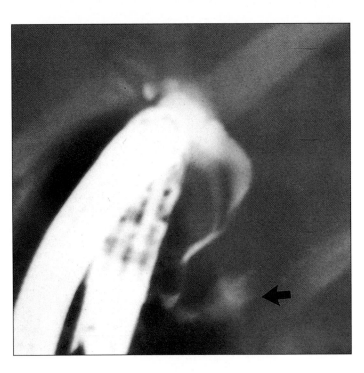

FIGURE 6-8.

Acinarization of the ventral pancreas during endoscopic retrograde cholangiopancreatography (*arrow*). This degree of acinarization is not clinically important, but recognition of this finding and the need to focus attention on the minor papilla are emphasized.

TABLE 6-4. TIPS TO MINOR PAPILLA CANNULATION

Long endoscope position is preferred

Total cessation of peristalsis required using glucagon or anticholinergics

Gentle technique is required to avoid trauma to minor papilla

Having correct tools available (*see* Fig. 6-9) is essential

Use of secretin to identify the orifice may be required

TABLE 6-4.

Tips to minor papilla cannulation [15–18].

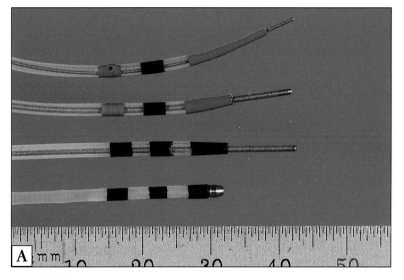
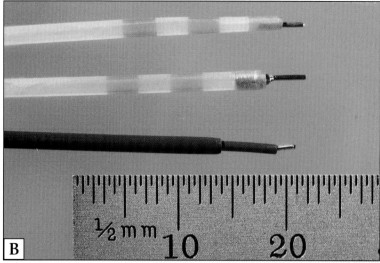

FIGURE 6-9.

Cannulation devices. **A,** Four 5-Fr diameter catheters commonly used for endoscopic retrograde cholangiopancreatography. Top: Highly tapered long nose with 0.018″ diameter guidewire, especially for the minor papillae. An extra side hole has been added at the proximal color band to permit air to escape during wire exchanges. Middle: Two slightly tapered tip catheters with 0.035″ diameter guidewires. Bottom: Metal ball-tipped catheter. The latter three are generally used for work on the major papillae. **B,** Top and Middle: 23-gauge needle-tipped catheters. The short needle tip is generally preferred. Bottom: 0.018″ diameter guidewire within 3-Fr catheter, which is within a 5-Fr catheter.

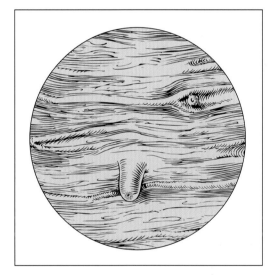

FIGURE 6-10.

Diagram showing endoscopic view of medial aspect of descending duodenum. The minor papilla is typically located approximately 2 cm cephalad and 1 to 2 cm anterior (right) of the major papilla. Valvulae conniventes occasionally deviate around the minor papilla as shown.

TABLE 6-5. USE OF SECRETIN TO FACILITATE MINOR PAPILLA CANNULATION

TABLE 6-5.

Use of secretin to facilitate minor papilla cannulation.

Needed in approximately one third of cases

Dosage of 0.5–1 unit per kg given intravenously as bolus.
Rapid juice flow generally precludes ability to inject contrast media to the tail

Only transient obstruction of the orifice with guidewires and catheters is permitted during active secretory phase, because excessive intraductal pressure may arise

Spraying methylene blue onto the minor papilla helps to identify the orifice during secretory juice flow

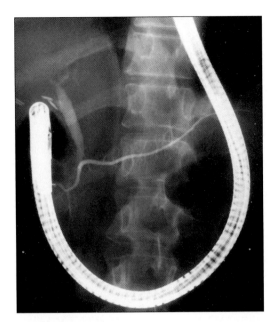

FIGURE 6-11.

Typical normal dorsal ductogram. This is very similar to a standard ductogram obtained through the major papilla. The endoscope is in the long position. The common bile duct is only partially filled.

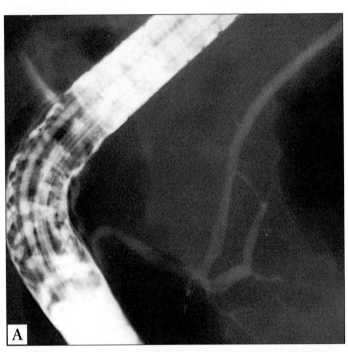

FIGURE 6-12.

A, Incomplete pancreas divisum. Note the main duct narrowing over a 5-mm length as it joins the dorsal duct. This narrowing must be differentiated from a pathologic stricture, as is seen with cancer. **B,** Dorsal ductogram obtained through the minor papilla that shows diffuse changes of chronic pancreatitis. The arrow in the lower left corner indicates a tiny ansa ventral branch that connects to the major papilla (*ie*, incomplete pancreas divisum).

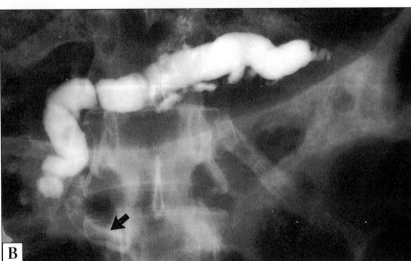

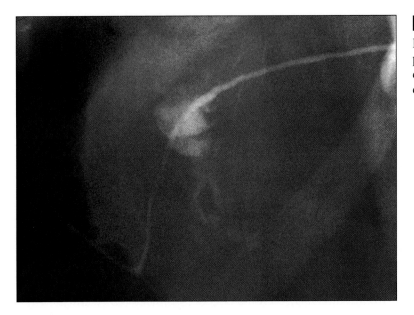

FIGURE 6-13.

Dorsal ductogram obtained through the minor papilla, which shows pseudocyst filling from near genu. The dorsal duct in the head is diffusely narrowed from compression by the pseudocyst and adjacent inflammation.

TABLE 6-6. OPTIONS FOR MANAGEMENT OF PATIENTS WITH PANCREAS DIVISUM

TABLE 6-6.

Options for management of patients with pancreas divisum [19–24].

Ignore if this variant anatomy appears clinically irrelevant (*eg*, patients with gallstone)

Medical therapy (oral pancreatic enzyme supplements and secretory suppression with anticholinergics)

Endoscopic therapy (stent with or without sphincterotomy)

Surgical therapy (sphincteroplasty)

Pancreatitis complication management (*eg*, pseudocysts, stones, strictures)

TABLE 6-7. OBSERVATIONS IMPLYING THAT MINOR PAPILLA NARROWING IS CAUSING OBSTRUCTION TO OUTFLOW OF DORSAL PANCREATIC JUICE

TABLE 6-7.

Observations implying that minor papilla narrowing is causing obstruction to outflow of dorsal pancreatic juice [25–31].

Chronic pancreatitis or duct dilation of the dorsal gland coexistent with a normal ventral gland

Prolonged dilation of the dorsal duct after intravenous secretin, as monitored by ultrasonography

Cystic dilation of the terminal dorsal duct (Santorinicele)

Probes and guidewires greater than 30/1000" diameter will not pass easily into the minor papilla without significant resistance

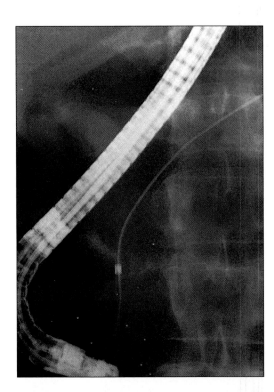

FIGURE 6-14.

Stent placement in the minor papilla. A guidewire has been passed to the tail of the pancreas. A 5-Fr, 2.5-cm length stent has been passed into the minor papilla.

TABLE 6-8. MINOR PAPILLA STENTING IN PATIENTS WITH PANCREAS DIVISUM WITH RECURRENT PANCREATITIS

	STENT (*n*=10)	CONTROL (*n*=10)	P
Hospital visits	0	7	< 0.05
Episodes of pancreatitis	0	7	< 0.05
Overall improvement	9/10	1/9	< 0.05

TABLE 6-8.

Data from randomized, controlled trial of endoscopic minor papilla stenting for a 1-year interval (stents exchanged at 3- to 4-month intervals). Stenting largely eliminated pancreatitis. (*Adapted from* Lans *et al.* [32].)

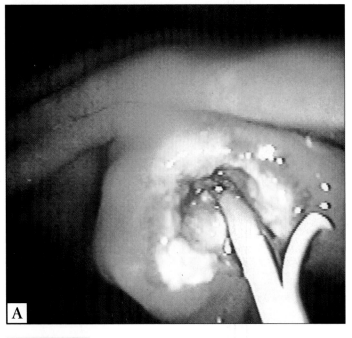

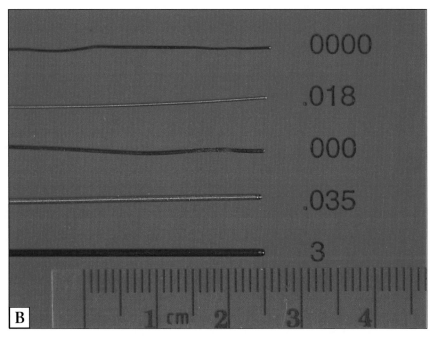

FIGURE 6-15.

Minor papilla view after needle knife sphincterotomy. **A,** A 5-Fr stent has been placed into the minor papilla; the tissue of the minor papilla has been incised with cautery with a needle knife. **B,** Dilating and sizing probes for intraoperative use in sphincter evaluations. Top to bottom: 4-0 lacrimal probe; 0.018″ diameter endoscopic retrograde cholangiopancreatography (ERCP) guidewire (for comparison); 3-0 lacrimal probe; 0.035″ diameter ERCP guidewire (for comparison); 3 Bakes dilator. (**A,** *Courtesy of* Stuart Sherman, Indiana University Medical Center.)

TABLE 6-9. PANCREAS DIVISUM: SURGICAL THERAPY OF MINOR PAPILLA

Author	Yr	Total, n	Patients Improved, %*	Recurrent Acute Pancreatitis		Pain Alone†		Re-stenosis	Major Complications	Deaths
				n	Patients Improved, %	n	Patients Improved, %			
Warshaw [13]	90	88	77	43	82	45	56	7/88	1/88	0
Brenner	90	13	54	10	70	3	0	0/13	0/13	0
Cooperman [31]	82	4	75	4	75	0	0	1/4	NG	0
Bragg [21]	88	4	100	3	100	1	100	0/4	NG	0
Rusnak	88	4	75	NG	—	NG	—	1/4	0/4	0
Madura [28]	86	32	75	11	82	19	68	NG	3/32	0
Britt	83	5‡	60	4	75	0	0	1/5	NG	0
Russell [19]	84	7	71	NG	—	NG	—	1/7	NG	0
Gregg [27]	83	19	53	NG	—	NG	—	1/19	1/19	1
Keith [20]	89	22‡	86	13	100	8	75	1/22	2/22	0
Totals	—	198	146/198 (74%)	73/88	83	45/76	59	14/166 (8%)	7/170 (4%)	0.5%

*Includes patients graded excellent, good, and fair (if > 50% improved and off narcotics).
†Pain suggestive of pancreatic origin (generally epigastric with back radiation) without serologic, ultrasound, computed tomographic, or ductographic evidence of pancreatitis.
‡Plus one patient with identification of failed minor papilla at laparotomy.
NG—not given.
All series used sphincteroplasty, except Keith, who used sphincterotomy.

TABLE 6-9. Pancreas divisum: surgical therapy of minor papilla.

TABLE 6-10. PANCREAS DIVISUM: ENDOSCOPIC SPHINCTEROTOMY THERAPY TO MINOR PAPILLA

Author	Yr	Total, n	Patients Improved, %	Recurrent Acute Pancreatitis		Pain Alone*		Chronic Pancreatitis		Re-stenosis	Major Complications	Deaths
				n	Patients Improved, %	n	Patients Improved, %	n	Patients Improved, %			
Soehenda	86	6	6/6 (100%)	2/2	100	—	—	4/4	100	—	0	0
Russell [19]	84	5†	1/5 (20%)	—	—	—	—	—	—	—	0	(1†)
Coleman [33]	93	13	7/13 (54%)	3/4	75	0	0	4/9	44	—	0	0
Lehman [37]	93	51	22/51 (43%)*	13/17	76	6/23	26	3/11	27	10/51	2/51	1§
Liguory [36]	86	8	5/8 (62%)	5/8	63	—	—	—	—	3/8	0	0
Totals	—	82	47/90 (52%)	23/31	74	6/23	26	11/24	46	13/59	2/83	1/83

*Includes only asymptomatic patients or those with minimal residual symptoms
†Five sphincterotomies achieved in 12 patients attempted
‡Death after Whipple's procedure (after failed endoscopic therapy)
§Minor papilla cannulation and therapy failed

TABLE 6-10. Pancreas divisum: endoscopic sphincterotomy therapy to minor papilla [33–37].

TABLE 6-11. COMPLICATIONS OF ENDOSCOPIC AND SURGICAL THERAPY TO MINOR PAPILLA

Complications from endoscopic stenting are less than from sphincterotomy

Mild pancreatitis is common

Stent-induced ductal changes are common and remain a significant concern

Endoscopic and surgical complication rates are similar

Major complications of serious pancreatitis or abscess occur in 2%–4% of patients; approximately 0.5%–1% death rates are reported

Because of the serious complication rates given here, therapy should be reserved for patients with recurrent pancreatitis or disabling pain

TABLE 6-11.

Complications of endoscopic and surgical therapy to minor papilla [38–41].

TABLE 6-12. MINOR PAPILLA THERAPY

PATIENTS WHO RESPONDED		PATIENTS WHO DID NOT RESPOND
✔	Acute recurrent pancreatitis	
	Chronic pancreatitis	✔
	Pain syndrome	✔
✔	Intermittent pain	
	Pain daily	✔
✔	Positive result to secretin ultrasound test	
✔	Lacrimal probe resistance	
✔	Dilated terminal dorsal duct	

TABLE 6-12.

Summary of symptomatic patients who are likely or unlikely to respond to minor papilla therapy.

ECTOPIC PANCREAS

TABLE 6-13. ECTOPIC PANCREAS

Ectopic islands of pancreatic tissue may occur almost anywhere in the gastointestinal tract

Present in approximately 2% of autopsy specimens

Rarely symptomatic

Usually submucosa

Most commonly located in gastric antrum, with central dimple representing rudimentary duct

Rarely give rise to neoplasm or focal pancreatitis

TABLE 6-13.

Ectopic pancreas [42,43].

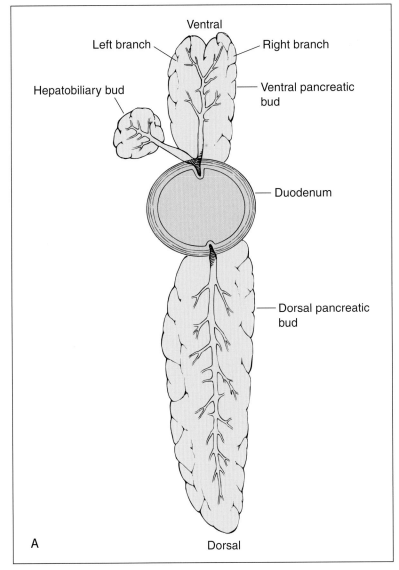

Ventral

Left branch — Right branch

Hepatobiliary bud — Ventral pancreatic bud

Duodenum

Dorsal pancreatic bud

A — Dorsal

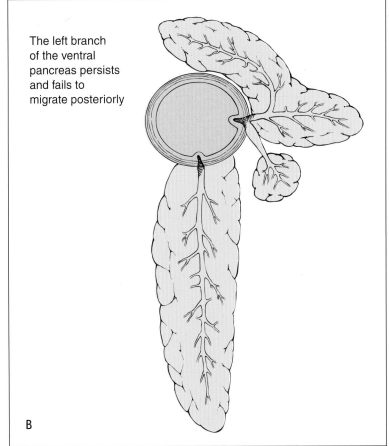

The left branch of the ventral pancreas persists and fails to migrate posteriorly

B

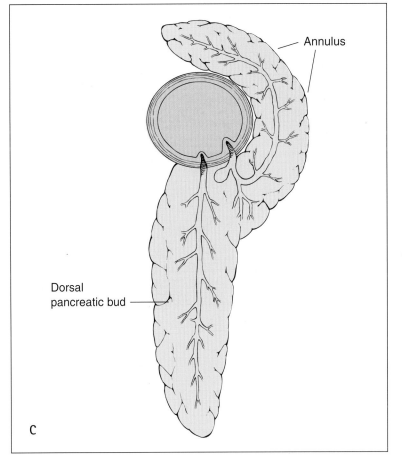

Annulus

Dorsal pancreatic bud

C

FIGURE 6-16.

Embryology of annular pancreas. Arises from faulty embryologic rotation of the ventral pancreas and/or persistence of the left ventral bud. It is seen in approximately 1 in 5000 autopsies, but up to 1 in 1000 endoscopic retrograde cholangiopancreatographies. The ring of tissue partially surrounds the descending duodenum in 75% of cases and completely surrounds the duodenum in 25% of cases. The minor papilla is invariably in the cephalad rim of the ring, and the major papilla is on the distal side. It mainly causes symptoms by descending duodenal narrowing. In approximately 10% of cases, the lesion is associated with pancreatitis. Duodenal bypass surgery is the preferred therapy. Approximately one third of the cases are associated with pancreas divisum. Fine-cut computed tomography or endoscopic ultrasound should also be diagnostic [44–50]. A, Same as Figure 6-1A, except left and right branches of ventral bud are labeled. B, Partial posterior ventral bud rotation has occurred. The left bud tip is adherent to its origin and is elongating. C, The dorsal and ventral parenchyma have fused, but ductal fusion has not yet occurred. The annulus surrounds the duodenum posteriorly.

(*continued on next page*)

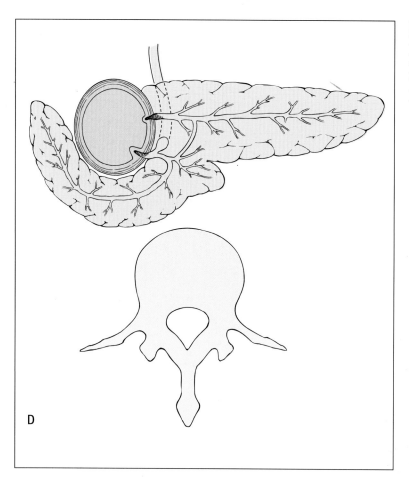

FIGURE 6-16. (CONTINUED)

D, A view as would be seen by CT scan in an adult. Ductal and parenchymal fusion has occurred. The annular pancreas surrounds the posterior wall of the descending duodenum. Duodenal luminal narrowing invariably occurs, but is not shown here.

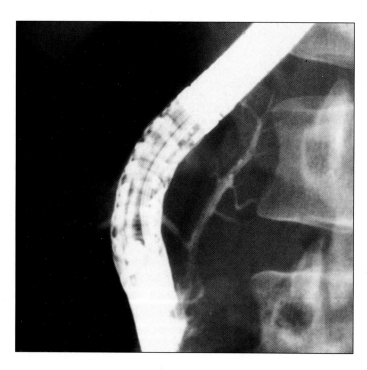

FIGURE 6-17.

Major papilla pancreatogram shows ventral pancreas (of pancreas divisum) combined with annular pancreas. Note branch encircling the endoscope and the descending duodenum. The result of the dorsal pancreatogram was normal.

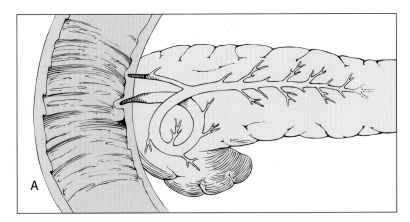

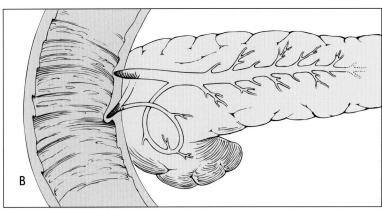

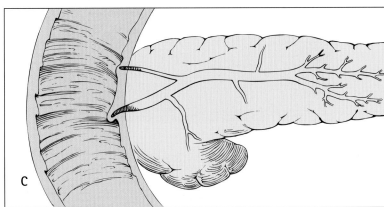

FIGURE 6-18.

A, Spiral (loop) contour in the head is the most common. **B,** Ansa pancreatica is second most common. Most of these are not clinically significant. A small-caliber ansa branch arising from the ventral pancreas is equivalent to incomplete pancreas divisum and is a variant of it. This atypical configuration may appear as pancreas enlargement by computed tomographic scan. **C,** Bifid tail [53,54].

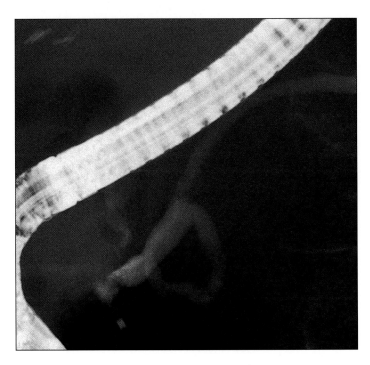

FIGURE 6-19.

Loop contour of main pancreatic duct. This was a coincidental finding in a patient with gallstones.

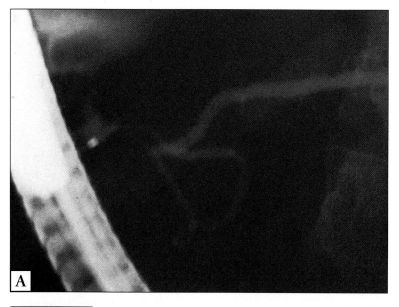

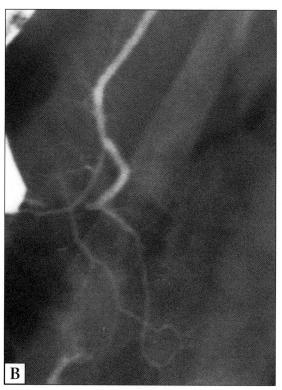

FIGURE 6-20.

Ansa pancreatica. **A**, The main duct has a ventral looping contour. This finding is generally of no clinical significance. **B**, Long branches extend into uncinate process from the main and accessory ducts. This finding is a normal variant.

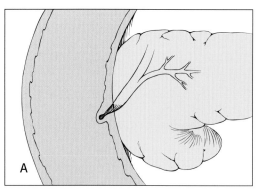

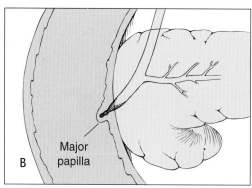

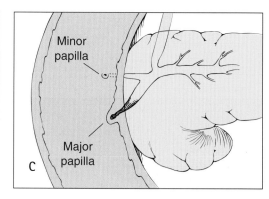

FIGURE 6-21.

Anomalous pancreatobiliary junction. By definition, anomalous pancreatobiliary junction occurs when the common channel is longer than 15 mm, thereby leaving the pancreatobiliary junction upstream from the sphincter of Oddi. Juice from the two ductal systems may intermix or variably be secreted into the alternative duct. This is thought to give rise to pancreatitis or choledochocele. **A**, Long common channel. **B**, The pancreatic duct appears to join the bile duct; the minor papilla is absent. **C**, The bile duct appears to connect into the pancreatic ductal system [55–57].

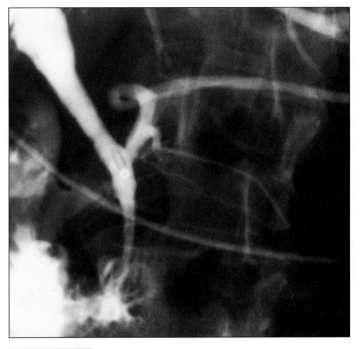

FIGURE 6-22.

Pancreatogram showing anomalous pancreatobiliary junction with simultaneous filling of the bile duct and pancreas from common channel injection. The common channel is 17 mm long.

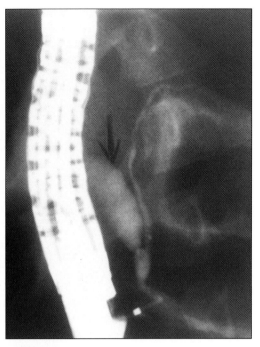

FIGURE 6-23.

Pancreatogram of anomalous pancreatobiliary junction associated with choledochal cyst and low-grade stricture at the downstream edge of the choledochal cyst.

TABLE 6-14. THERAPY OF ANOMALOUS PANCREATOBILIARY JUNCTION

Sphincterotomy or sphincteroplasty is recommended for such patients with pancreatitis

Surgical resection is generally recommended for extrahepatic choledochal cysts because they have a frequency for cholangiocarcinoma of approximately 10%

TABLE 6-14.

Therapy of anomalous pancreatobiliary junction.

■ ROLE OF CONGENITAL ANOMALIES IN IDIOPATHIC PANCREATITIS

TABLE 6-15. IDIOPATHIC ACUTE RECURRENT PANCREATITIS

ENDOSCOPIC RETROGRADE CHOLANGIOPANCREATOGRAPHY, SOM FINDINGS	VENU (n=116), %	SHERMAN (n=55), %	TOTAL (n=17), %
SO Dysfunction	15	33	20
Pancreas Divisum	10	15	11
Duct Stones	7	6	6
Choledochocele	3	4	4
Tumor (malignant/benign)	3	5	4
Total Abnormal	38	72	46

TABLE 6-15.

Lesions causing pancreatitis of otherwise unknown etiology. This table shows the findings in two such series. Although most patients did not have congenital anomalies, developmental anomalies are present in the differential diagnosis in this setting [62,63]. ERCP—endoscopic retrograde cholangiopancreatography; SO—sphincter of Oddi; SOM—sphincter of Oddi manometry.

REFERENCES

1. Tagge EP, Smith SD, Raschbaum GR, *et al.*: Pancreatic ductal abnormalities in children. *Surgery* 1991, 110:709–717.

2. Lemmel T, Hawes R, Sherman S, *et al.*: Endoscopic evaluation and therapy of recurrent pancreatitis and pancreaticobiliary pain in the pediatric population (abstract). *Gastrointest Endosc* 1993, 39:317A.

3. Putnam PE, Kocoshis SA, Oresenstein SR, Schade RR: Pediatric endoscopic retrograde cholangiography. *Am J Gastroenterol* 1991, 86:824–830.

4. Wagner CW, Golladay ES: Pancreas divisum and pancreatitis in children. *Am Surg* 1988, 54:22–26.

5. Quinlan RM: Anatomy and embryology of the pancreas. In *Shackelford's Surgery of the Alimentary Tract.* Edited by Turcotte J. Philadelphia: W.B. Saunders; 1991.

6. Narisawa R, Asakura H, Niwa M, Ogoshi K: Morphological study of the pancreas divisum using ERP in Niigata. *Digestive Endoscopy* 1993, in press.

7. Smanio T: Proposed nomenclature and classification of the human pancreatic ducts and duodenal papillae: Study based on 200 post mortems. *Int Surg* 1969, 52:125–134.

8. Cotton PB: Pancreas divisum: Curiosity or culprit (editorial)? *Gastroenterology* 1985, 89:1431–1435.

9. Tulassay Z, Papp J: New clinical aspects of pancreas divisum. *Gastrointest Endosc* 1980, 26:143–146.

10. Barton P, Person B, Charneau J, Boyer J: Pancreas divisum: A coincidental association. *Endoscopy* 1991, 23:55–58.

11. Carr-Locke DL: Pancreas divisum: The controversy goes on? *Endoscopy* 1991, 23:88–90.

12. Delhaye M, Engelholm L, Cremer M: Pancreas divisum: Congenital anatomic variant or anomaly? Contribution of endoscopic retrograde dorsal pancreatography. *Gastroenterology* 1985, 89:951–958.

13. Warshaw AL, Simeone JF, Schapiro RH, Flavin-Warsha B: Evaluation and treatment of the dominant dorsal duct syndrome (pancreas divisum redefined). *Am J Surg* 1990, 159:59–66.

14. Staritz M, Meyer zum Büschenfelde KH: Elevated pressure in the dorsal part of pancreas divisum: The cause of chronic pancreatitis? *Pancreas* 1988, 3:108–110.

15. Dunham F, Deltenre M, Jeanmart J, *et al.*: Special catheters for E.R.C.P. *Endoscopy* 1981, 13:81–85.

16. O'Connor KW, Lehman GA: An improved technique for accessory papilla cannulation in pancreas divisum. *Gastrointest Endosc* 1985, 31:13–17.

17. Schleinitz PF, Katon RM: Blunt tipped needle catheter for cannulation of the minor papilla. *Gastrointest Endosc* 1984, 30:263–266.

18. Benage D, McHenry R, Hawes R, *et al.*: Minor papilla cannulation and dorsal ductography in pancreas divisum. *Gastrointest Endosc* 1990, 36:553–557.

19. Russell RCG, Wong NW, Cotton PB: Accessory sphincterotomy (endocopic and surgical) in patients with pancreas divisum. *Br J Surg* 1984, 71:954–957.

20. Keith RG, Shapero TF, Sailbil FG, Moore TL: Dorsal duct sphincterotomy is effective long-term treatment of acute pancreatitis associated with pancreas divisum. *Surgery* 1989, 106:660–666.

21. Bragg LE, Thompson JS, Burnett DA: Surgical treatment of pancreatitis associated with pancreas divisum. *Nebr Med J* 1988:169–173.

22. Lowes JR, Rode J, Lees WR, *et al.*: Obstructive pancreatitis: Unusual causes of chronic pancreatitis. *Br J Surg* 1988, 75:1129–1130.

23. Siegel JH, Ben-Zvi JS, Pullano W, Cooperman A: Effectiveness of endoscopic drainage for pancreas divisum: Endoscopic and surgical results in 31 patients. *Endoscopy* 1990, 22:129–133.

24. McCarthy J, Geenen JE, Hogan W: Preliminary experience with endoscopic stent placement in benign pancreatic diseases. *Gastrointest Endosc* 1988, 34:16–18.

25. Foley TR, McGarrity TJ: Transient changes of dorsal pancreatic duct in acute pancreatitis associated with pancreas divisum. *Dig Dis Sci* 1990, 35:793–797.

26. Blair AJ, Russell CG, Cotton PB: Resection for pancreatitis with pancreas divisum. *Am Surg* 1984, 200:590–594.

27. Gregg JA, Monaco AP, McDermott WV: Pancreas divisum: results of surgical intervention. *Am J Surg* 1983, 145:488–492.

28. Madura JA, Fiore AC, O'Connor KW, *et al.*: Pancreas divisum: Detection and management. *Am Surg* 1985, 51:353–357.

29. Madura JA: Pancreas divisum: Stenosis of the dorsally dominant pancreatic duct. *Am J Surg* 1986, 151:742–745.

30. Traverso LW, Musser G, Peer WW, *et al.*: Pancreas divisum: The role of pancreatic ductal drainage. *Surg Gastroenterol* 1982, 1:11–16.

31. Cooperman M, Ferrara JJ, Fromkes JJ, Carey LC: Surgical management of pancreas divisum. *Am J Surg* 1982, 143:107–112.

32. Lans JI, Geenen JE, Johanson JF, Hogan WJ: Endoscopic therapy of patients with pancreas divisum and acute pancreatitis: A prospective randomized controlled trial. *Gastrointest Endosc* 1992, 38:430–434.

33. Coleman SD, Eisen GM, Troughton AB, Cotton PB: Endoscopic treatment in pancreas divisum. *Am J Gastroenterol* 1994, 89:1152–1155.

34. Soehendra N, Kempeneers I, Nam VCH, Grimm H: Endoscopic dilatation and papillotomy of the accessory papilla and internal drainage. *Endoscopy* 1986, 18:129–132.

35. Chevillotte G, Sahel J, Pietri H, Sarles H: Pancréatites aiguës à rechutes, associées au pancréas divisum: Étude clinique de 12 cas. *Gastroenterol Clin Biol* 1984, 8:352–358.

36. Liguory C, Lefebvre JF, Canard JM, *et al.*: Le pancréas divisum: étude clinique et thérapeutique chez l'homme: a propos de 87 cas. *Gastroenterol Clin Biol* 1986, 10:820–825.

37. Lehman GA, Sherman S, Nisi R, Hawes R: Pancreas divisum: Results of minor papilla sphincterotomy. *Gastrointest Endosc* 1993, 39:1–8.

38. Kozarek RA: Pancreatic stents can induce ductal changes consistent with chronic pancreatitis. *Gastrointest Endosc* 1990, 36:93–95.

39. Burdick JS, Geenen JE, Johanson JF, *et al.*: Morphologic predictors of response to stent therapy in chronic pancreatitis (abstract). *Am J Gastroenterol* 1992, 87:1281.

40. Smith M, Ikenberry S, Uzer M, *et al.*: Alterations in pancreatic ductal morphology following pancreatic stent therapy (abstract). *Gastrointest Endosc* 1993, 39:332.

41. Sherman S, Alvarez C, Rober M, *et al.*: Polyethylene pancreatic duct stent-induced changes in the normal dog pancreas. *Gastrointest Endosc* 1993, 39:657–664.

42. Dolan RV, ReMine WH, Dockerty MB: The fate of heterotopic pancreatic tissue: A study of 212 cases. *Arch Surg* 1974, 109:762–765.

43. Jeng KS, Yang KC, Juo SHF: Malignant degeneration of heterotopic pancreas. *Gastrointest Endosc* 1991, 37:196–198.

44. Gilmore PR, Agarwal VP: Endoscopic evaluation of heterotopic pancreas (case report). *Gastrointest Endosc* 1989, 35:563–565.

45. Dowsett JF, Rode J, Russell RCG: Annular pancreas: A clinical, endoscopic, and immunohistochemical study (case study). *Gut* 1989, 30:130–135.

46. Yogi Y, Shibue T, Hashimoto S: Annular pancreas detected in adults, diagnosed by endoscopic retrograde cholangiopancreatography: Report of four cases (case report). *Gastroenterol Jpn* 1987, 22:92–99.

47. Itoh Y, Hada T, Terano A, *et al.*: Pancreatitis in the annulus of annular pancreas demonstrated by the combined use of computed tomography and endoscopic retrograde cholangiopancreatography. *Am J Gastroenterol* 1989, 84:961–964.

48. Gilinsky NH, Lewis JW, Flueck JA, Fried AM: Annular pancreas associated with diffuse chronic pancreatitis. *Am J Gastroenterol* 1987, 82:681–684.

49. Sperrazza JC, Flanagan RA, Katlic MR: Annular pancreas and intermittent duodenal obstruction in an alcoholic adult. *Clev Clin J Med* 1992, 59:206–210.

50. Lehman GA, O'Connor KW: Coexistence of annular pancreas and pancreas divisum–ERCP diagnosis. *Gastrointest Endosc* 1985, 31:25–28.

51. Nishimori I, Okazaki K, Morita M, *et al.*: Congenital hypoplasia of the dorsal pancreas: With special reference to duodenal papillary dysfunction. *Am J Gastroenterol* 1990, 85:1029–1033.

52. Wildling R, Schnedl WJ, Reisinger EC, *et al.*: Agenesis of the dorsal pancreas in a woman with diabetes mellitus and in both of her sons. *Gastroenterolgy* 1993, 104: in press.

53. Halpert RH, Shabot JM, Heare BR, Rogers RE: The biphid pancreas: A rare anatomical variation. *Gastrointest Endosc* 1990, 36:60–61.

54. Yatto RP, Siegel JH: Variant pancreatography. *Am J Gastroenterol* 1983, 78:115–118.

55. Misra SP, Dwivedi M: Pancreatobiliary ductal union. *Gut* 1990, 31:1144–1149.

56. Mori K, Nagakawa T, Ohta T, *et al.*: Acute pancreatitis associated with anomalous union of the pancreaticobiliary ductal system. *J Clin Gastroenterol* 1991, 13:673–677.

57. Ng WT, Wong MK, Chan YT, Liu K: Clinical application of the study on sphincter of Oddi motor activity in patients with anomalous pancreatobiliary junction. *Am J Gastroenterol* 1992, 87:926–927.

58. Ikoma A, Nakamura N, Miyazaki T, Maeda M: Double cancer of the gallbladder and common bile duct associated with anomalous junction of pancreaticobiliary ductal system. *Surgery* 1992, 111:595–600.

59. Ueda N, Nagakawa T, Ohta T, *et al.*: Synchronous cancer of the biliary tract and pancreas associated with anomalous arrangement of the pancreaticobiliary ductal system. *J Clin Gastroenterol* 1992, 15:136–141.

60. Miyazaki K, Date K, Imamura S, *et al.*: Familial occurrence of anomalous pancreaticobiliary duct union associated with gallbladder neoplasms. *Am J Gastroenterol* 1989, 84:176–181.

61. Howard JM: Cysts of the pancreas. In *Surgical disease of the pancreas*. Edited by Howard JM, Jordan GL, Reber HA. Philadelphia: Lea & Febiger; 1987.

62. Venu RP, Geenen JE, Hogan W, *et al.*: Idiopathic recurrent pancreatitis: An approach to diagnosis and treatment. *Dig Dis Sci* 1989, 34:56–60.

63. Sherman S, Jamidar P, Reber H: Idiopathic acute pancreatitis (IAP): Endoscopic approach to diagnosis and therapy. *Gastrointest Endosc* 1993, 39:331.

Chapter 7

Pancreatic Carcinoma

. . . .

Pancreatic cancer is a highly lethal clinical entity whose frequency has been increasing over the years. Its incidence is now ninth among cancers not associated with skin, and it is the fourth most common cause of death from cancer. It makes up about 3% of all cancers and causes about 6% of all cancer deaths. Almost 95% of all patients afflicted with this disease eventually die from it (compared with only 80% in lung cancer). The incidence increases with age, as more than 80% of all patients are older than 60; it is more common in men than in women. Racial factors may also play a role. Blacks in the United States have one of the highest risks for pancreatic cancer in the world, with a 30% to 40% higher risk than whites. There is also a higher incidence in developed countries.

Few definitive risk factors for pancreatic cancer have been identified other than cigarette smoking, which can increase the relative risk up to five times. Other possible associations with environmental factors are not yet firmly defined. Most pancreatic cancers are adenocarcinomas; however, many different histologic types of pancreatic cancer exist. The importance of these differences is not well defined. The cancer itself has often spread to local or distant organs by the time of presentation. Metastases are found, in descending order of frequency, in the liver, regional lymph nodes, peritoneum, and lungs, in up to 85% of all patients with the disease.

The best hope for cure in patients with pancreatic cancer depends on early diagnosis. Signs or symptoms, however, often do not develop until late in the disease, after metastases have occurred. Pancreatic carcinoma often presents in a nonspecific manner. The classic triad of weight loss, abdominal or back pain, and jaundice is seen frequently. Many other symptoms (*eg*, malaise, nausea, anorexia), however, are nonspecific and commonly seen in other clinical conditions. For this reason, diagnosis may be delayed in some patients.

Jaundice is one of the most frequent physical signs of pancreatic cancer; it occurs when the cancer obstructs the bile duct.

MARK T. TOYAMA
AMY M. KUSSKE
HOWARD A. REBER

Other physical signs that may be present include hepatomegaly and a palpable gallbladder (ie, Courvoisier's gallbladder). Diagnosis of pancreatic cancer has been approached differently at various institutions. Recently, however, the approach has become more or less standardized. A wide array of diagnostic tests is available; a combination of two or three is usually the best approach. The work-up usually starts with noninvasive tests and progresses to more sophisticated and invasive studies as the diagnosis becomes more likely.

Noninvasive studies that have been used in the diagnosis include upper gastrointestinal series, abdominal ultrasound, and computed tomography (CT). CT scanning is the best diagnostic test and provides the most important information in most cases.

Invasive studies include endoscopic retrograde cholangiopancreatography (ERCP), percutaneous cholangiography, and percutaneous or endoscopic biopsy or brushing. These have less important roles in the initial diagnosis than computed tomography scans, but they can offer important additional information in special circumstances.

Biochemical markers that have been studied as potential aids in the diagnosis of pancreatic cancer include presence of carcinoembryonic antigen, pancreatic oncofetal antigen, and a variety of monoclonal antibodies. The most widely used currently is cancer antigen 19-9, which correlates with tumor burden. Therapy for pancreatic carcinoma has changed over the years as endoscopic technology has improved with more experience. The use of both percutaneous and endoscopic stents has eliminated the need for operation in some patients with pancreatic cancer. Patients who are reasonable operative risks and have potentially resectable disease, however, should undergo laparotomy after appropriate work-up has ruled out distant metastases.

The standard operative treatment for resectable pancreatic carcinoma is Whipple's pancreaticoduodenectomy. This operation involves resection of the pancreatic head, antrum of the stomach, duodenum, and distal common bile duct. Functional anatomy is restored by a hepaticojejunostomy, gastrojejunostomy, and pancreaticojejunostomy. A variation of this procedure is the pylorus-sparing pancreaticoduodenectomy. This procedure is the same as the standard Whipple, but does not involve resection of the stomach and pylorus. Proponents believe that this option results in better gastric function postoperatively. Opponents argue that it may not be an adequate cancer operation. Further evaluation and study are needed to resolve this controversy. Although total pancreatectomy has been used in the past, the morbidity and operative mortality rates were higher than with the standard Whipple, and long-term survival was no better. Therefore, it is rarely used today.

The morbidity and mortality rates of the Whipple operation have improved dramatically. Morbidity is now about 15% and mortality is less than 5% in experienced hands; however, the long-term survival rate after a Whipple operation is only about 10%. One recent study had an encouraging 5-year survival rate of 18%.

Palliation of patients with unresectable pancreatic cancer and obstructive jaundice has been accomplished with a biliary intestinal bypass, often accompanied by a gastrojejunostomy to palliate gastric outlet obstruction; however, recent improvements in percutaneous and endoscopic biliary stent technology have permitted nonoperative palliation in some patients.

Survival rates in patients who undergo an attempted curative resection are influenced by the degree of tumor differentiation and the presence or absence of lymph node metastases. Patients with well-differentiated tumors and negative findings in the lymph nodes have the best survival rates.

Medical options in the treatment of pancreatic cancer are limited, and survival is usually less than 1 year. Treatment options include radiotherapy, chemotherapy, hormonal therapy, immunotherapy, and combinations of these, with or without surgery. The best chance for patients with pancreatic carcinoma is found with early diagnosis and curative operative resection.

TABLE 7-1. EPIDEMIOLOGIC CHARACTERISTICS OF PANCREATIC CANCER

FACTORS ASSOCIATED WITH INCREASED RISK OF PANCREATIC CANCER

Age
Male sex
Greatest among blacks in U.S.
Urban setting
Low socioeconomic class
Tobacco smoking
Alcohol consumption (?)
Pancreatitis
Coffee consumption
Tea consumption
Dietary factors
  Meat consumption
  Fat consumption
Occupational factors
  Radiation exposure
  Chemical exposure
Previous history of gastrectomy
Diabetes

FACTORS ASSOCIATED WITH A DECREASED RISK OF PANCREATIC CANCER

Fruit and vegetable consumption
Allergic disease
Tonsillectomy

TABLE 7-1.

Although specific causes have not yet been elucidated, a variety of factors are associated with the development of pancreatic cancer. Age-specific incidence rates show that the disease is uncommon before age 45 and increases steadily thereafter. More than 80% of all cases occur in the 60- to 80-year-old age group; it is more common in males. A variety of dietary factors, such as a high consumption of fat, low consumption of fruit and vegetables, and high coffee and alcohol consumption, have been potentially linked to pancreatic cancer development. The strongest epidemiologic association is with tobacco consumption, where there is a two- to threefold increased risk of development. The mechanism by which tobacco consumption increases the risk of pancreatic cancer is unclear. It is possible that carcinogens in the smoke are secreted in bile, reflux into the pancreatic duct from the duodenum, or reach the pancreas through the bloodstream [1,2].

TABLE 7-2. HISTOLOGIC CLASSIFICATION OF EXOCRINE PANCREATIC TUMORS

Ductal cell origin
  Ductal cell carcinoma
  Giant cell carcinoma
  Giant cell carcinoma
    Osteoclastoid
  Adenosquamous carcinoma
    Spindle-cell carcinoma
  Microadenocarcinoma
  Mucinous carcinoma
  Mucinous cystadenocarcinoma
  Papillary cystic tumor
  Mucinous carcinoid carcinoma
  Carcinoid
  Oncocytic carcinoid
  Oncocytic carcinoma
  "Oat cell" carcinoma
  Ciliated cell carcinoma
Acinar cell origin
  Acinar-cell carcinoma
  Acinar cystadenocarcinoma
Uncertain histogenesis
  Pancreaticoblastoma (simple)
  Pancreaticoblastoma (mixed type)
  Unclassified
    Small-cell carcinoma
    Large-cell carcinoma
    Clear -cell carcinoma
Mixed cell type
  Duct-islet-cell carcinoma
  Duct-islet-acinar-cell carcinoma
  Acinar-islet-cell carcinoma
  Carcinoid-islet-cell carcinoma
Connective tissue origin
  Leiomyosarcoma
  Malignant fibrous histiocytoma
  Hemangiopericytoma
  Fibrosarcoma
  Malignant neurilemoma

TABLE 7-2.

Histologic classification system for exocrine pancreatic tumors. This system is based on the histologic and submicroscopic appearance of the tumors. The most common type of pancreatic cancer is ductal-cell carcinoma, with an incidence of 70% to 80% in most series [2a].

HISTOLOGY

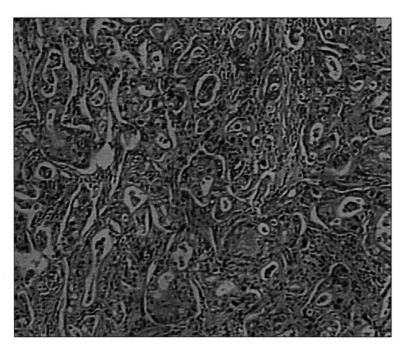

FIGURE 7-1.

Ductal cell carcinoma. These tumors tend to occur in the head of the pancreas; only about one third are located in the body or tail. Tumors in the head are usually smaller than those in the body or tail. The size of the tumor does not necessarily correlate with the grade of malignancy, however. The tumors often originate from the epithelium of the main pancreatic duct branches, and may produce irregular strictures and chronic pancreatitis distal to the stricture. Microscopically, these tumors demonstrate an absence of zymogen and neurosecretory granules in most cells and a tubular ductal arrangement of the tumor cells. Other cellular characteristics seen are loss of polarity, nuclear polymorphism, prominent nucleoli, and enlarged nuclei. There is also typically a highly desmoplastic reaction of the surrounding stroma.

SYMPTOMS

TABLE 7-3. PRESENTING SYMPTOMS IN PANCREATIC CARCINOMA

SYMPTOM	PATIENTS, %
Weight loss	91
Pain	83
Jaundice	71
Anorexia, nausea	44
Malaise	34
Vomiting	13

TABLE 7-3.

The three most common symptoms of pancreatic cancer are weight loss, pain, and jaundice [3]. The weight loss that occurs may be quite severe (*ie*, up to 10 kg). The greater and the more rapid the loss, the greater is the likelihood that the tumor will *not* be resectable. Painless jaundice, often regarded as a classical presenting symptom, is actually relatively uncommon [4]. Pain alone is usually dull and located in the mide-pigastrium. Depending on the location and spread of the tumor, the pain may radiate to the back or either subcostal area. A persistent back-ache can signify retroperitoneal invasion and a very poor prognosis. Jaundice, when it occurs, is often the symptom that initiates a patient's evaluation. Periampullary tumors often present with jaundice relatively early, and therefore have a better rate of cure; however, jaundice occurring with body or tail tumors can signify hepatic or hilar metastases, and therefore inoperability. Uncommon symptoms or findings include migratory thrombophlebitis, sciatica (caused by retroperitoneal nerve infiltration), or enlarged supraclavicular (Virchow's) or periumbilical (Sister Mary Joseph's) nodes. (*Adapted from* Trede and Carter [3]; with permission.)

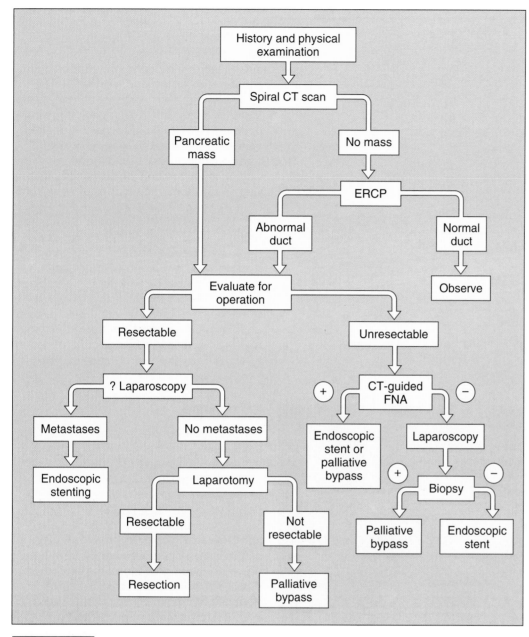

FIGURE 7-2.

When the history and physical examination suggest the possibility of pancreatic cancer, the first diagnostic test the authors use a spiral computed tomography (CT) scan. If a pancreatic mass is detected, then the patient is evaluated for operation. If no mass is seen on CT scan, then the

patient will undergo an endoscopic retrograde cholangiopancreatography (ERCP). If the ERCP demonstrates normal pancreatic and common bile ducts, then the patient may be observed with close follow-up. If the duct anatomy is abnormal, then the patient is evaluated for operation. Some endoscopists may also obtain endoscopic needle aspiration or duct brushings at this point as well.

Patients are evaluated for operation on the basis of CT evidence for resectability and presence of metastases. If the CT scan demonstrates metastases or definite involvement of the major vessels (*eg*, portal vein or superior mesenteric artery) by tumor, the patient's diseases are classified as unresectable. Other factors that may influence whether or not a patient is an operative candidate are their ages and general overall medical condition.

In patients determined to be candidates for operation, the use of laparoscopy as a first step is controversial. Advocates perform laparoscopy to determine if there are any peritoneal or liver metastases present that were not detected by the CT scan. If metastases are present, laparotomy is avoided and the patient may undergo endoscopic stenting. If no metastases are detected by laparoscopy, the patient will undergo laparotomy. Intraoperative determination of resectability will then determine whether or not the patient is a candidate for a resection of the tumor or a palliative bypass procedure. If a patient is *not* an operative candidate, tissue confirmation of pancreatic cancer is the next step; this is done using CT- or ultrasound-guided fine-needle aspiration (FNA). Endoscopic FNA, biopsy, or brushings are also options. If the biopsy is positive, then the patient can undergo endoscopic stenting or be reevaluated for a palliative bypass. If the biopsy is negative, the patient can undergo laparoscopy and biopsy.

TABLE 7-4. DIAGNOSTIC WORK-UP FOR PANCREATIC CANCER: LABORATORY FINDINGS

Elevated bilirubin

Elevated liver function tests

Elevated alkaline phosphatase

Elevated serum blood sugar

Elevated amylase

Occult blood in the stool

Low hemoglobin

Tumor markers

    Gastrointestinal cancer-associated antigen (CA 19-9)

    Carcinoembryonic antigen (CEA)

    CA-50

    α-fetoprotein (AFP)

    Pancreatic oncofetal antigen (POA)

Genetic markers

    p52

    K-*ras*

TABLE 7-4.

Diagnostic work-up. There are no good laboratory tests for pancreatic cancer. Often, the cancer has progressed too far by the time it produces abnormal laboratory values. When the cancer obstructs the common bile duct, significant elevations in serum bilirubin and liver function tests can occur [5]. The other findings, such as elevated blood sugar levels (possibly due to islet cell dysfunction or destruction), elevated amylase levels (from pancreatic cell destruction), or signs and symptoms of chronic blood loss, occur with varying frequency and are nonspecific [6]. Certain tumor markers may improve the detection of pancreatic cancer. Cancer antigen 19-9 correlates fairly well with tumor burden; high values indicate a larger tumor or disseminated disease. More recently, genetic markers have been proposed as possible means to detect early pancreatic cancer. They could be detected in malignant cells obtained by duodenal intubation or in the stool. Their usefulness has yet to be determined, but they may provide a relatively easy and accurate means of early detection in some cases.

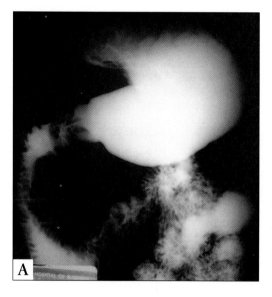

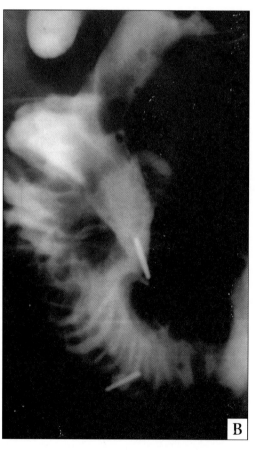

FIGURE 7-3.

Barium studies of the gastrointestinal (GI) tract are not often used to evaluate patients with suspected pancreatic cancer. Because many of these patients present with nonspecific gastrointestinal symptoms, however, an upper GI may be obtained. Findings on upper GI that suggest pancreatic cancer include extrinsic compression, displacement or encasement of the C-loop, mucosal invasion (nodularity or spiculation), or Frostberg's reversed '3' sign. **A,** Widened duodenal sweep and the suggestion of compression of part of the duodenal loop. **B,** Note the reversed '3' sign caused by the nodular compression of the medial duodenal wall by the pancreatic cancer. (*Courtesy of* Dr. Barbara Kadell, UCLA Department of Radiology.)

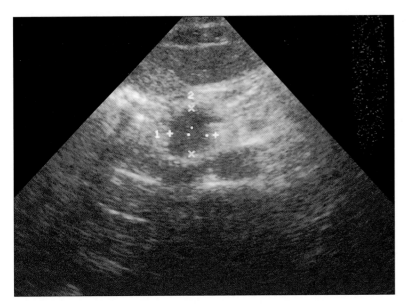

FIGURE 7-4.

Ultrasound can be a useful diagnostic modality to evaluate a patient with jaundice of unknown etiology. If the cause of the jaundice is biliary obstruction from a pancreatic tumor, the extra- and intrahepatic bile ducts are dilated. If the cause of the jaundice is intrahepatic, the ducts are of normal diameter. Ultrasound is inferior to computed tomography scanning both for tumor detection and staging of the disease. It is therefore not recommended for screening if pancreatic cancer is strongly suspected.

Angiography

TABLE 7-5. DIAGNOSTIC WORK-UP OF PANCREATIC CANCER: ANGIOGRAPHY

Findings on angiography in pancreatic carcinoma	Also useful for
Hypovascular mass	Definition of vascular anatomy
Encasement of intrapancreatic vessels	Identification of vascular anomalies that could complicate pancreatic resection
Encasement of extrapancreatic arteries and veins (indicative of unresectability)	Origin of hepatic artery from superior mesenteric artery
	Nonmalignant obstruction of major arteries

TABLE 7-5.

Angiography can be used to detect vascular involvement of a pancreatic tumor. It can also define the peripancreatic vascular anatomy before operation. With the advent of spiral computed tomography (CT) scans, however, definition of the peripancreatic vasculature is good and determination of resectability can often be made on the basis of CT scan alone. Therefore, angiography has no role in the evaluation of a patient with suspected pancreatic carcinoma.

Computed tomography

TABLE 7-6. DIAGNOSTIC WORK-UP OF PANCREATIC CANCER: CT SCAN

Findings of CT scans in pancreatic carcinoma	Criteria for determination of resectability
Focal or diffuse mass in the pancreas; usually decreased attenuation of the mass relative to normal pancreas	Local extension of tumor
Biliary duct obstruction	Invasion of contiguous organs
Intra- and extrahepatic	Vascular involvement
Gallbladder distension	Metastases
Pancreatic duct obstruction	Hepatic
Ascites	Lymph node
	Other (distant)

TABLE 7-6.

Computed tomography (CT) scans are the most accurate method to diagnose and stage pancreatic cancer. The findings of pancreatic carcinoma that can be seen on CT scan are listed in this table. In addition, CT scans can determine whether or not a patient's tumor is resectable based on the criteria listed.

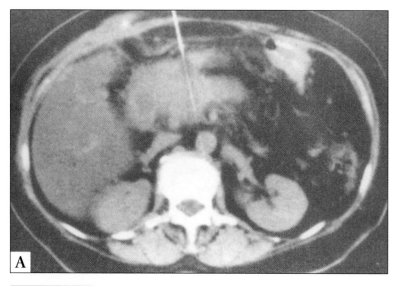
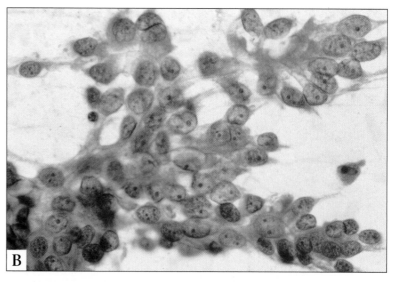

FIGURE 7-5.

A, Computed tomography (CT) can also direct a needle aspiration to obtain a tissue diagnosis from a pancreatic mass. **B,** Atypical cells, as seen on this CT-guided needle aspiration sample, signify the presence of pancreatic carcinoma. This procedure plays an important role in patients who are not operative candidates either because their tumors are not resectable or they are in poor medical condition. Confirmation of pancreatic cancer with tissue involvement can initiate palliative procedures, such as endoscopic stenting, chemotherapy, or reevaluation for an operative bypass. (*Courtesy of Dr. Barbara Kadell, UCLA Department of Radiology.*)

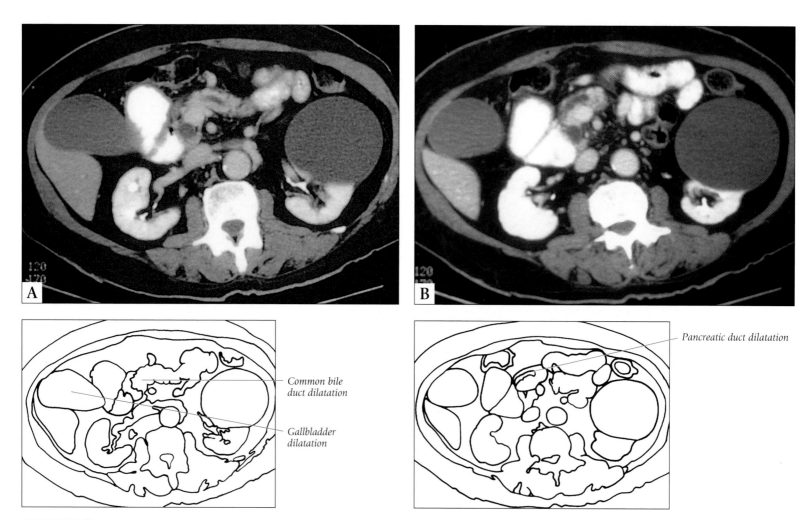

FIGURE 7-6.

A–B, Computed tomography scans demonstrating common bile duct and gallbladder dilatation (**panel A**); pancreatic duct dilatation is also evident (**panel B**). **C,** Mass in the head of the

(continued on next page)

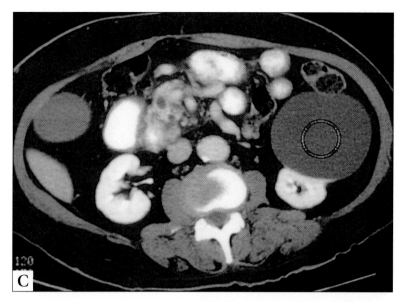

C

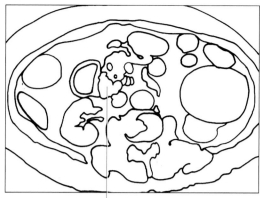

Mass in the head of the pancreas

FIGURE 7-6. (CONTINUED)

pancreas. Note the presence of a left renal cyst in all three panels. (*Courtesy of* Dr. Barbara Kadell, UCLA Department of Radiology.)

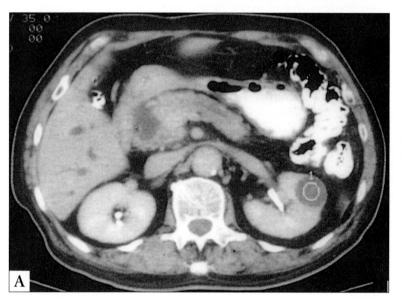

A

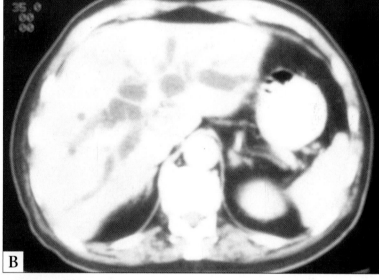

B

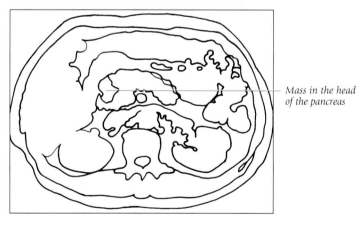

Mass in the head of the pancreas

FIGURE 7-7.

A, Computed tomography scan demonstrating a mass in the head of the pancreas. B, Massive intrahepatic biliary dilatation secondary to obstruction of the common bile duct resulting from the pancreatic tumor. (*Courtesy of* Dr. Barbara Kadell, UCLA Department of Radiology.)

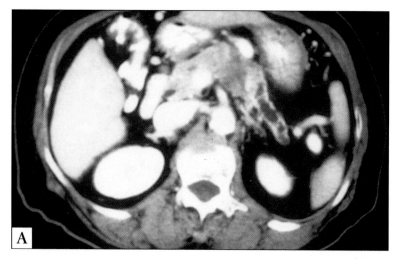

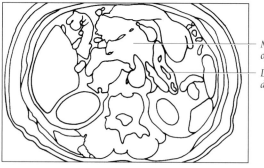

Mass in the body
of the pancreas

Dilated pancreatic
duct

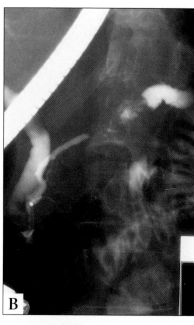

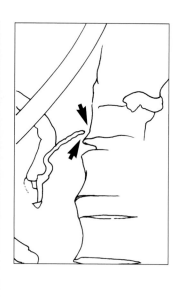

FIGURE 7-8.

A, Computed tomography scan demonstrates a mass in the body
of the pancreas with a dilated pancreatic duct distal to the mass.
B, Endoscopic retrograde cholangiopancreatography in the same
patient showing a stricture (between arrows) in the pancreatic duct
with significant distal pancreatic duct dilatation. (*Courtesy of* Dr.
Barbara Kadell, UCLA Department of Radiology.)

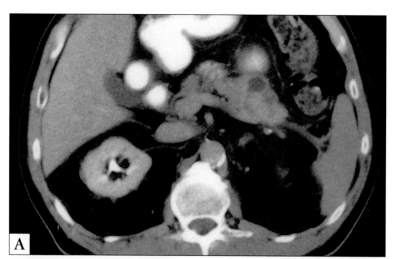

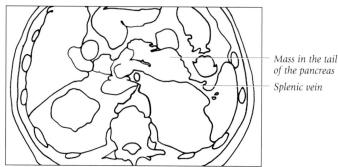

Mass in the tail
of the pancreas

Splenic vein

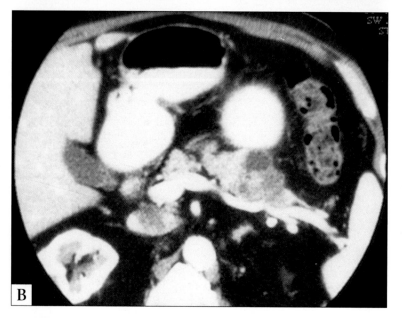

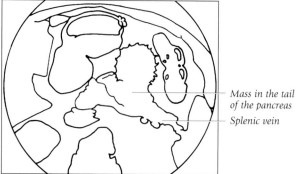

Mass in the tail
of the pancreas

Splenic vein

FIGURE 7-9.

A, Spiral computed tomography scan demonstrating a mass in the
tail of the pancreas. **B**, Close-up view demonstrates adherence of
the mass to the splenic vein. (*Courtesy of* Dr. Barbara Kadell, UCLA
Department of Radiology.)

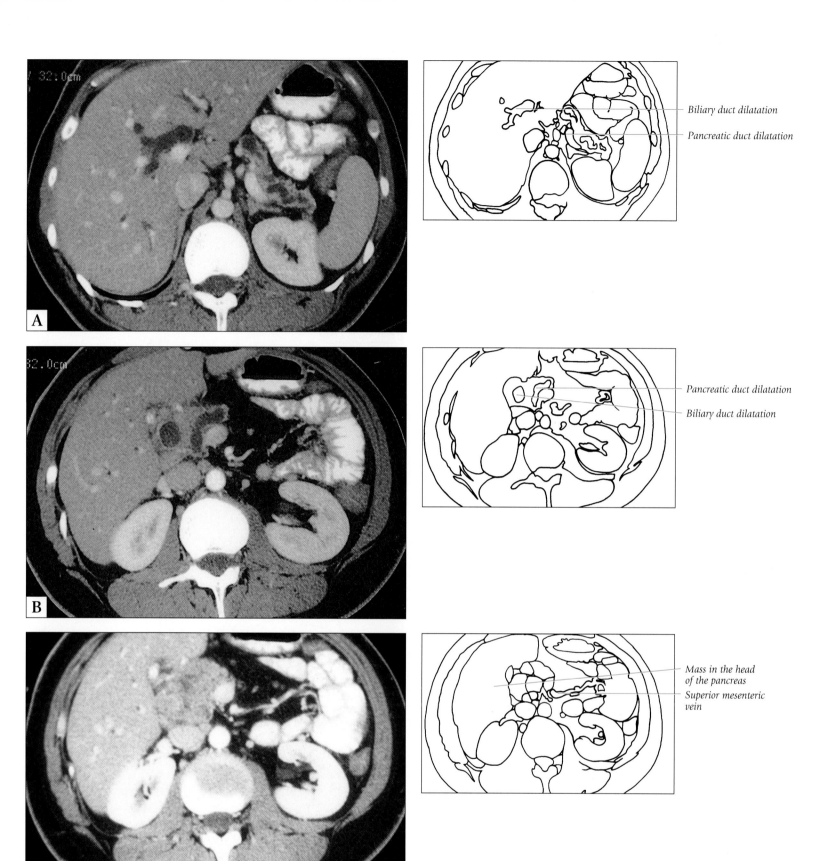

FIGURE 7-10.

A, Computed tomography scan demonstrates intrahepatic biliary duct and pancreatic duct dilatation. **B,** Extrahepatic bile duct and pancreatic duct dilation. **C,** Mass in the head of the pancreas, which appears contiguous with the superior mesenteric vein.

At operation the patient was found to have a tumor invading the superior mesenteric vein, which was unresectable for that reason. (*Courtesy of* Dr. Barbara Kadell, UCLA Department of Radiology.)

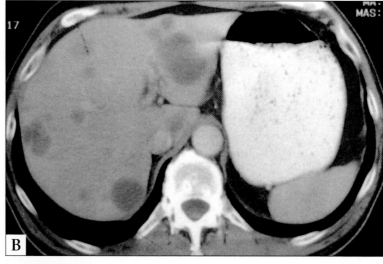

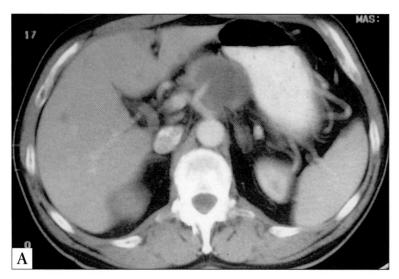

*Mass in the head
of the pancreas*

*Superior mesenteric
artery*

FIGURE 7-11.

A, Computed tomography (CT) scan demonstrates encasement of the superior mesenteric artery by a mass in the head of the pancreas. **B,** CT scan of the liver in the same patient showing the presence of multiple liver metastases. This patient's tumors would not be resectable because of involvement of a major vascular structure and the presence of metastatic disease. (*Courtesy of* Dr. Barbara Kadell, UCLA Department of Radiology.)

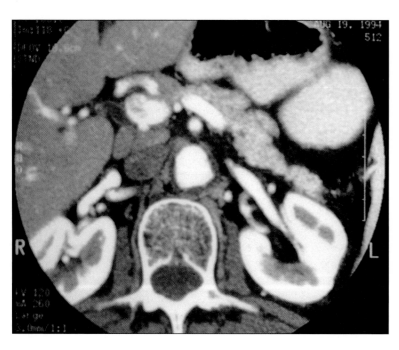

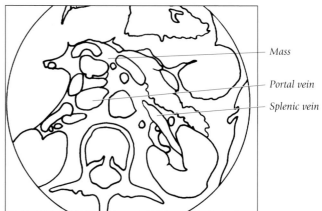

Mass

Portal vein

Splenic vein

FIGURE 7-12.

This close-up view of a spiral computed tomography scan shows a mass involving the portal vein and splenic vein. This patient also would not be resectable because of tumor involvement of major vascular structures. (*Courtesy of* Dr. Barbara Kadell, UCLA Department of Radiology.)

TABLE 7-7. DIAGNOSTIC WORK-UP OF PANCREATIC CANCER: ENDOSCOPIC RETROGRADE CHOLANGIOPANCREATOGRAPHY

Findings of ERCP in pancreatic carcinoma

Endoscopy

    Mass bulging into the stomach or duodenum

    Direct visualization of tumor eroding into the gut lumen

Cholangiopancreatography

    Obstruction of the pancreatic or common bile duct

    Disruption or stenosis of the pancreatic duct with or without prestenotic ectasia

    Displacement of the pancreatic or common bile duct

    Acinar or field defects

    Pooling of contrast secondary to duct necrosis and tumor cavitation

    Double duct sign: Stricture of the bile and pancreatic ducts at the same level with upstream dilatation. This is a classic finding in many patients with pancreatic cancer.

TABLE 7-7.

Diagnostic work-up of pancreatic cancer: endoscopic retrograde cholangiopancreatography (ERCP).

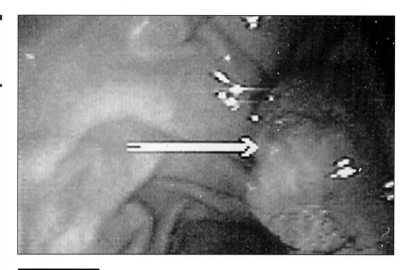

FIGURE 7-13.

Endoscopic view of a pancreatic carcinoma that has grown into the duodenum and is visible on endoscopy (*arrow*). Biopsies of masses such as this one are easy to obtain to confirm the diagnosis; however, even if endoscopic retrograde cholangiopancreatography demonstrates this finding and tissue biopsy confirms pancreatic carcinoma, a computed tomography scan remains necessary to determine whether or not the pancreatic mass is potentially resectable.

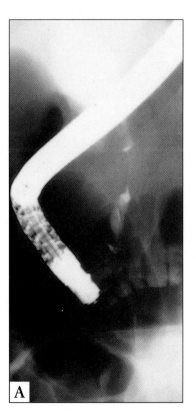
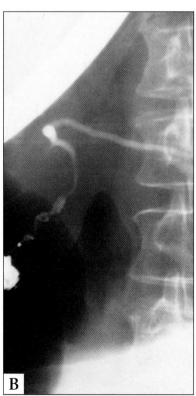

FIGURE 7-14.

A, Endoscopic retrograde cholangiopancreatography demonstrating a narrowed intrapancreatic segment of common bile duct. **B,** Pancreatogram in the same patient demonstrating displacement and narrowing of the pancreatic duct within the head of the pancreas.

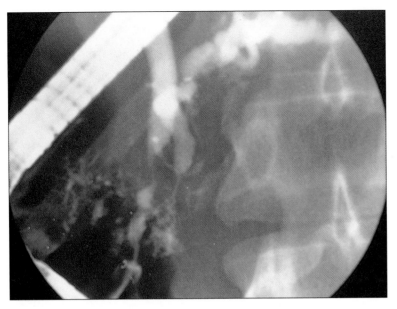

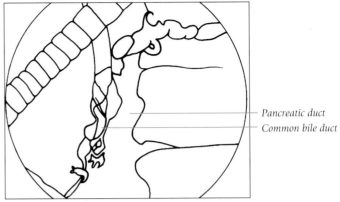

FIGURE 7-15.

Endoscopic retrograde cholangiopancreatography demonstrating the "double duct" sign. Note the narrowing of both the common bile duct and pancreatic duct at the same level within the head of the pancreas, and the distal dilatation in the pancreatic duct.

FIGURE 7-16.

Endoscopic retrograde cholangiopancreatography demonstrating biopsy of an intrapancreatic biliary duct stricture. The film shows endoscopic biopsy forceps being passed into the duct to obtain tissue for histologic evaluation. Endoscopy can provide several ways to obtain pancreatic tissue in cases of suspected cancer, including forceps biopsy, needle biopsy, needle aspiration, or intraductal brushings.

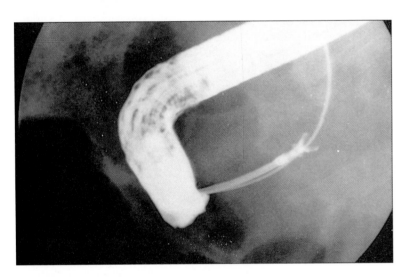

Transhepatic cholangiography

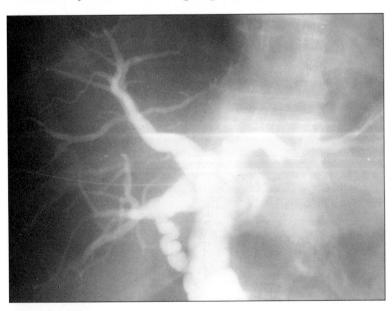

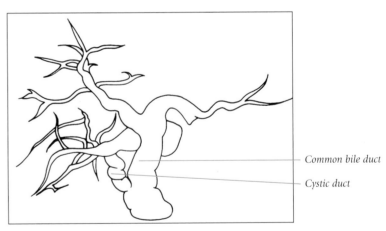

FIGURE 7-17.

Transhepatic cholangiogram demonstrating complete obstruction of the common bile duct below the level of the cystic duct with marked proximal intra- and extrahepatic biliary dilatation. Transhepatic cholangiogram is rarely used as a primary diagnostic study. Endoscopic retrograde cholangiopancreatography can often delineate abnormal biliary duct anatomy. When the common bile duct is completely obstructed, however, transhepatic cholangiograms can further define the obstruction and provide access to the biliary tree for drainage if needed.

Whipple's operation

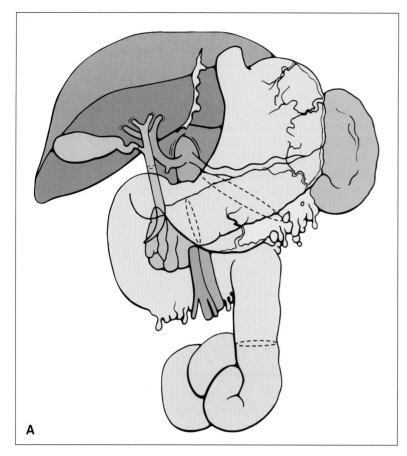

A

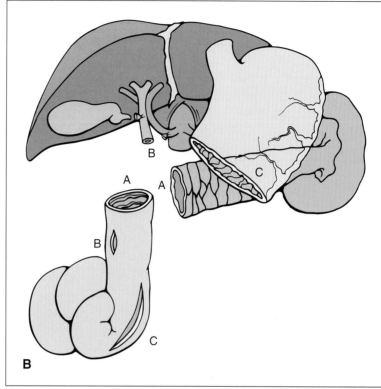

B

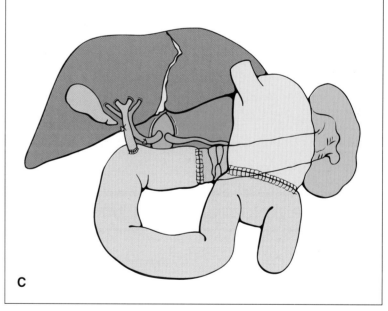

C

FIGURE 7-18.

The standard Whipple operation, which involves resection of the common bile duct, the gallbladder, the duodenum, and the pancreas to the level of the midbody. **A,** Lines of resection. **B,** Anatomy after resection and before reconstruction (A-A—pancreaticojejunostomy; B-B—choledochojejunostomy; C-C—gastrojejunostomy). **C,** Anatomy after reconstruction.

Pancreatic resection for pancreatic cancer is appropriate only if all gross tumor can be removed with standard resection. The lesion is considered resectable if the following areas are free of tumor: the hepatic artery near the origin of the gastroduodenal artery; the portal and superior mesenteric veins as they pass in front of the uncinate process and behind the body of the pancreas; the superior mesenteric artery, where it courses under the body of the pancreas; and the liver and regional lymph nodes. About 20% of cancers of the head of the pancreas can be resected, but because of local and distant spread, this is rarely possible for lesions of the body and tail. (*Adapted from* Reber [6a].)

Pancreatoduodenectomy (pylorus-sparing)

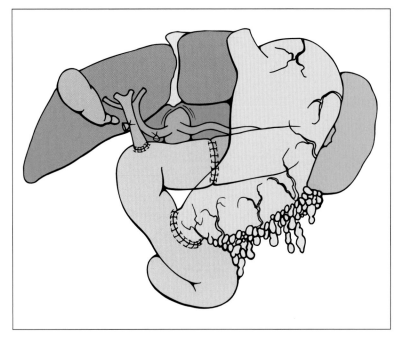

FIGURE 7-19.

Reconstruction after a pancreatoduodenectomy that preserved the pylorus. Instead of the antrectomy that is done with the standard Whipple, the stomach, including the pylorus, is preserved and reanastomosed with the jejunum. This operation was designed as an alternative to the standard Whipple. Many of its proponents argue that it is "more physiologic," therefore patients would have fewer gastrointestinal complaints and nutritional deficits postoperatively compared with the Whipple. No randomized prospective trails have shown this to be true, however. Some believe that this operation may not be adequate when used for malignant tumors, and that the standard Whipple should be performed for all pancreatic cancers. (*Adapted from* Reber [6a].)

■ MORTALITY RATES

TABLE 7-8. OPERATIVE MORTALITY OF WHIPPLE OPERATION FOR CANCER

AUTHOR	INSTITUTION	PATIENTS, NO.	OPERATIVE MORTALITY (%)
van Heerden *et al.* [5]	Mayo Clinic	146	6 (4.1)
Jones *et al.* [6]	Toronto	87	4 (4.6)
Grace *et al.* [7]	UCLA	45	1 (2.2)
Bittner *et al.* [8]	Ulm	55	3 (5.4)
Pellegrini *et al.* [9]	University of California, San Francisco	51	1 (2.0)

TABLE 7-8.

Operative mortality of the Whipple operation from several institutions over time is shown. In experienced centers the Whipple operation can be done safely, with a lower than 4% mortality. (*Adapted from* Trede [4]; with permission.)

TABLE 7-9. LONG-TERM SURVIVAL RATES AFTER WHIPPLE OPERATION FOR CANCER

AUTHOR	INSTITUTION	PATIENTS, NO.	5-YR SURVIVAL RATE, %
Cooperman [10]	Columbia	70	7.1
van Heerden *et al.* [11]	Mayo Clinic	44	2.3
Jones *et al.* [6]	Toronto	28	7.0
Grace *et al.* [7]	UCLA	37	3.0
Connolly *et al.* [12]	University of Chicago	89	3.4
Crist and Cameron [13]	Johns Hopkins	50	18.0

TABLE 7-9.

As seen in the previous table, long-term survival rates for patients with pancreatic cancer remain approximately 5%. There is no difference in long-term survival between patients undergoing total pancreatectomy versus partial pancreatectomy; therefore, the Whipple operation remains preferable to more radical total pancreatectomy. (*Adapted from* Trede [4]; with permission.)

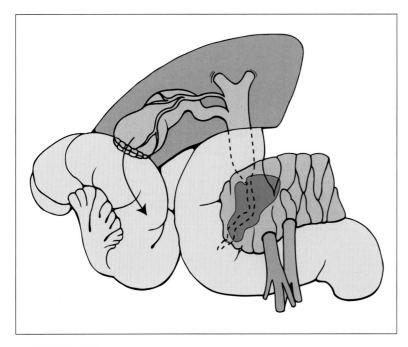

FIGURE 7-20.

A bypass operation done for unresectable pancreatic cancer. Biliary drainage is diverted through the gallbladder into the jejunum. The operation can be done with low operative morbidity and mortality rates; it provides relief from jaundice and pruritus. (*Adapted from* Reber [6a].)

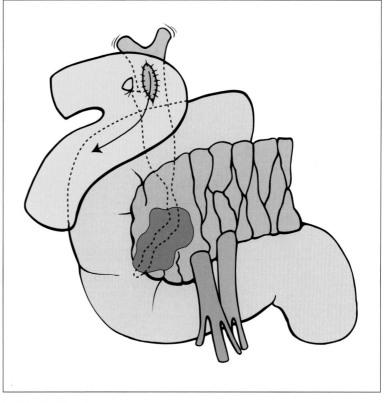

FIGURE 7-21.

Another type of bypass operation done for unresectable pancreatic cancer. This type of bypass is preferable when the cancer is near the cystic duct, which would cause a cholecystojejunostomy to obstruct eventually. It also provides relief from jaundice and pruritus. (*Adapted from* Reber [6a].)

FIGURE 7-22.

Gastrojejunostomy is required if the tumor blocks the duodenum. If laparotomy has been performed, many surgeons believe that gastrojejunostomy should be done prophylactically because with time, obstruction often develops before other life-threatening complications. (*Adapted from* Reber [6a].)

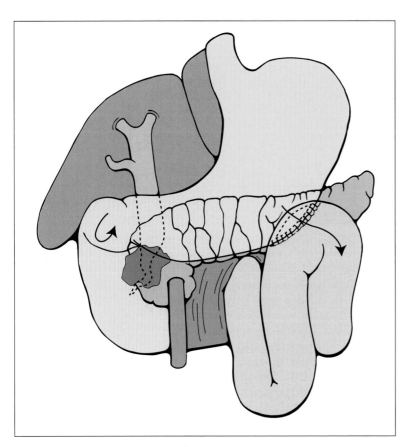

SURVIVAL RATES

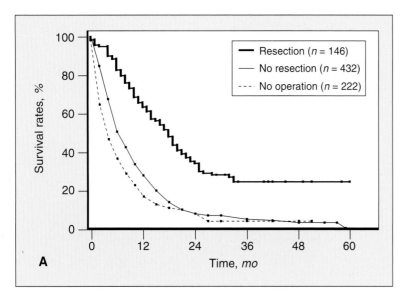

FIGURE 7-23.

A, Survival rates in patients with pancreatic carcinoma treated in various ways. **B,** Survival rates in patients with pancreatic carcinoma based on tumor differentiation. **C,** Survival rates in patients with pancreatic carcinoma based on the presence or absence of lymph node metastases [17]. These results demonstrate some important considerations in treatment. Overall survival rates are poor despite improvements in patient care; however, patients who had a resection had a significant improvement in 5-year survival rates. Tumor differentiation influenced survival as well. Those with poorly differentiated tumors had significantly worse survival rates than those with better differentiated tumors. This is not unexpected because the less differentiated tumors tend to be more aggressive, invasive, and resistant to therapy. The presence of lymph node metastases also influences the overall survival rate. (*Adapted from* Geer and Brennan [17]; with permission.)

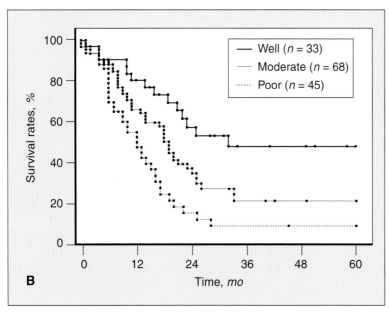

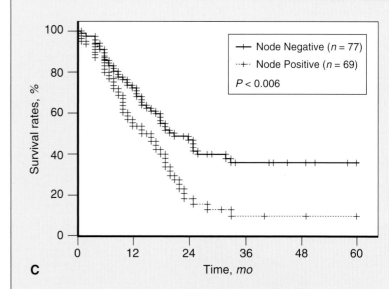

NONSURGICAL OPTIONS

TABLE 7-10. NONSURGICAL THERAPY OF PANCREATIC CARCINOMA: OPTIONS

Radiotherapy

External beam radiation of the upper abdomen, usually in conjunction with chemotherapy

Intraoperative radiation therapy—Iodine 125, usually in conjunction with chemotherapy and external beam radiation

Hormonal

Tamoxifen

Chemotherapy

5-fluorouracil

Combination chemotherapy

Immunotherapy

TABLE 7-10.

Medicotherapeutic options for the treatment of pancreatic carcinoma are limited. Local radiotherapy combined with chemotherapy (5-fluorouracil) has been shown in a study from the Gastrointestinal Tumor Study Group [18,19] to increase survival by 6 to 8 months. Long-term survival is unusual, but occasionally occurs. Pancreatic cancer has been considered to be relatively "radioresistant." Irradiation is made more difficult by the deep location of the pancreas and its proximity to areas that are sensitive to radiation (intestine, spinal cord, liver, kidneys).

Hormonal therapy has not been shown to be of value in unresectable pancreatic carcinoma. Although immunotherapy with monoclonal antibodies has shown some initially promising results, this treatment is new and requires further study.

CHEMOTHERAPEUTIC DRUGS

TABLE 7-11. SINGLE-AGENT CHEMOTHERAPY IN PANCREATIC CANCER

DRUG	RESPONSE RATE ±95%, CI
5-fluorouracil	28±6
Mitomycin-C	21±6
Streptozoticin	11±6
Methyl lomustine	4±2
BCNU (1,3-bis [2-chloroethyl]-1-nitrosurea)	0
Doxorubicin	7±5
Ifosfamide	12±6

TABLE 7-11.

Many anticancer drugs have been used to treat pancreatic cancer. Only 5-fluorouracil (5-FU) has a response rate with 95% confidence intervals greater than 20%. Although several agents have been used in combination regimens, their single-agent activity in pancreatic cancer is poor. In several uncontrolled trials the small numbers of patients made evaluation of response rates difficult. In general, the partial responses seen with single-agent therapy are brief and rarely associated with clinical benefit. Combination therapy was initially reported to increase response rates, but these findings have not been confirmed. Median survivals are still probably not better than those obtained with 5-FU alone. With the current inability to treat pancreatic cancer medically, more effective treatments are needed for all disease stages. These may evolve as understanding of the etiology, growth regulation, and drug resistance of pancreatic cancer increases. Gemcitabine is one of the newest agents currently being evaluated. The response rate is 5% to 10%; the median survival is 5.6 months; and 18% of the patients are still alive at 1 year; however, 24% of the patients reported being symptomatically improved with treatment. (*Adapted from* Arbuck [20]; with permission.)

REFERENCES

1. Fontham ETH, Correa P: Epidemiology of pancreatic cancer. *Surg Clin North Am* 1989, 69:551–567.

2. Boyle P, Hsieh CC, Maisonneuve P, *et al.*: Epidemiology of pancreas cancer. *Int J Pancreat* 1989, 5:327–346.

2a. Cubilla AL, Fitzgerald PF: Tumors of the exocrine pancreas. In *Atlas of Tumor Pathology*. Washington, DC: Armed Forces Institute of Pathology; 1984.

3. Trede M, Carter DC: Clinical evaluation and preoperative assessment. In *Surgery of the Pancreas*. Edited by Trede M, Carter DC. Edinburgh: Churchill Livingstone; 1993:423–431.

4. Trede M: The surgical options. In *Surgery of the Pancreas*. Edited by Trede M, Carter DC. Edinburgh: Churchill Livingstone; 1993:433–442.

5. van Heerden JA, McIlrath DC, Ilstrup DM, Weiland LH: Total pancreatectomy for ductal adenocarcinoma of the pancreas: An update. *World J Surg* 1988, 12:658–662.

6. Jones BA, Langer B, Taylor BR, Girotti M: Periampullary tumors: Which ones should be resected? *Am J Surg* 1987, 149:46–52.

6a. Reber HA: The pancreas. In *Principles of Surgery*, edn 6. Edited by Schwartz S. New York: McGraw-Hill; 1994.

7. Grace PA, Pitt HA, Longmire WP Jr: Pancreatoduodenectomy with pylorus preservation for adenocarcinoma of the head of the pancreas. *Br J Surg* 1986, 73:647–650.

8. Bittner R, Roscher R, Safi F, *et al.*: Der Einfluss von Tumorgrösse und Lymphknotenstatus auf die Prognose des Pankreaskarzinoms. *Chirurg* 1989, 60:240–245.

9. Pellegrini CA, Heck FC, Raper S, Way LW: An analysis of the reduced morbidity and mortality rates after pancreaticoduodenectomy. *Arch Surg* 1989, 124:778–781.

10. Cooperman AM: Cancer of the pancreas: A dilemma in treatment. *Surg Clin North Am* 1981, 61:107–115.

11. van Heerden JA, ReMine W, Weiland L, *et al.*: Total pancreatectomy for ductal adenocarcinoma of the pancreas. *Am J Surg* 1981, 142:308–311.

12. Connolly MM, Dawson PJ, Michelassi F, *et al.*: Survival in 1001 patients with carcinoma of the pancreas. *Ann Surg* 1987, 206:366–371.

13. Crist DW, Cameron JL: Current status of pancreaticoduodenectomy for periampullary carcinoma. *Hepatogastroenterology* 1989, 36:478–485.

14. Bakkevold KE, Arnesjo B, Kambestad B: Carcinoma of the pancreas and papilla of Vater: Presenting symptoms, signs, and diagnosis related to stage and tumour site. *Scand J Gastroenterol* 1992, 27:317–325.

15 Singh SM, Longmire WP, Reber HA: Surgical palliation for pancreatic cancer. *Ann Surg* 1990, 212:132–139.

16. Warren KW, Christophi C, Armendariz R, Basu S: Current trends in the diagnosis and treatment of carcinoma of the pancreas. *Am J Surg* 1983, 145:813–818.

17. Geer RJ, Brennan MF: Prognostic indicators for survival after resection of pancreatic adenocarcinoma. *Am J Surg* 1993, 165:68–72.

18. Moertel CG, Frytak S, Hahn RG, *et al.*: Therapy of locally unresectable pancreatic carcinoma. *Cancer* 1981, 48:1705–1710.

19. Kalser MH, Ellenberg SS: Pancreatic cancer: Adjuvant combined radiation and chemotherapy following curative resection. *Arch Surg* 1985, 120:899–903.

20. Arbuck SE: Overview of chemotherapy for pancreatic cancer. *Int J Pancreat* 1990, 7:209–222.

Chapter

8

Rationale and Application of Radioligand Imaging in Gastroenterology

RODNEY V. POZDERAC
THOMAS M. O'DORISIO

Beginning with the discovery and isolation of secretin from the canine gastrointestinal (GI) mucosa by Bayliss and Starling in 1902 [1], our understanding of the biochemistry, physiology, pathophysiology, and especially, the clinical significance of the regulatory gut peptide substances has grown at an astounding pace. Between 1986 and 1991 alone nearly 14,000 journal articles were published on GI peptides [2]. We have learned that many of these peptides have a variety of absorptive, secretory, digestive, motor, and trophic actions; trophic actions (*eg*, gastrin) work not only on the secretory, absorptive, and motility cells of the GI tract, but also on other endocrine and nonendocrine organ systems [2,3].

SOMATOSTATIN

One of the most important developments in the field of GI endocrinology and peptide research was the discovery and isolation of somatostatin in 1972 by Brazeau and colleagues [4], and the subsequent synthesis of the long-acting congener, octreotide acetate (SMS 201-995, Sandostatin). Somatostatin has been localized not only to the hypothalamus from which it was originally extracted, but also in the endocrine pancreas and in the whole neuroendocrine cell and peptidergic nervous system of the GI tract. It exists naturally as a ringed 28- or 14-amino acid residue structure. Further, somatostatin is known to function at various times as: (1) an endocrine peptide acting through the circulation; (2) a paracrine peptide acting next to its cell site of origin; (3) a neurocrine peptide acting through its release from peptidergic nerve endings onto its target cells; and (4) an autocrine peptide acting onto its own cell of origin [5]. Somatostatin exerts a tonic inhibition on the release of several pituitary peptides that include growth hormone (GH), adrenal corticotropin hormone (ACTH), prolactin (PRL), and thyroid-stimulating hormone (TSH) [6]. Somatostatin also inhibits the release of several intestinal peptides, including insulin, glucagon, motilin, glucose-dependent insulinotropic peptide (GIP), vasoactive intestinal peptide (VIP), secretin, cholecystokinin, and gastrin-releasing peptide (GRP) [6]. Extensive physiologic studies with somatostatin have demonstrated its antisecretory and proabsorptive gastrointestinal properties. It inhibits salivary, gastric, pancreatic, and biliary secretion as well [5]. (*see* Table 8-1.)

Somatostatin congeners

A number of powerful congeners (analogues) of somatostatin have been developed, and include the clinically approved octreotide acetate [7]. Other synthesized somatostatin congeners include lanreotide (BIM-23014C), RC-160, MK-678, and CGP-27996. These congeners have not yet been approved for clinical use in the United States. Figure 8-1 depicts the structure of native somatostatin and its congeners, octreotide and lanreotide. It can be noted that both congeners are ringed structures, like somatostatin, and both retain the Trp-Lys amino acid residues. The lysine residue is thought to be the important biologic binding unit of the peptide to its respective somatostatin receptor-positive cells.

The clinically approved congener, octreotide acetate, exerts powerful inhibitory and antagonistic action on regulatory peptide release and peptide-specific target cells. Table 8-3 lists octreotide's powerful effects and alludes to its present clinical use as well as its other potential clinical applications [8]. A consensus statement regarding octreotide's role in inhibiting some forms of severe secretory diarrhea was recently published [9]. The statement alludes to octreotide's broad-spectrum efficacy in secretory diarrheal states not necessarily related to the watery diarrhea syndrome of carcinoid or VIPoma, the latter of which is an indication approved by the Food and Drug Administration.

Radiolabeled somatostatin congener scintigraphy

The rationale and logical extension of somatostatin and its congeners' clinical application should to be further developed and reviewed, particularly as they relate to in situ, noninvasive scintigraphy. At the levels of both the endocrine organ and the tumor cell, somatostatin appears to inhibit signal transduction. Among the signal transduction pathways antagonized by somatostatin are the second-messenger formation of cyclic adenosine monophosphate (cAMP) [10], diacyel glycerol (DAG), ion channel action (Ca^{2+}, K^+) [11], and protein phosphorylation (tyrosine phosphatatse) activation [12]. The ability of one somatostatin to antagonize multiple signal transduction pathways suggested the possibility of more than a single subtype of somatostatin receptor. Recent studies describing and reviewing five somatostatin receptor subtypes and signal transduction action have been published [13]. A critically important publication demonstrating high-density somatostatin receptors on gastrointestinal and neuroendocrine tumors appeared in 1987 by Reubi and colleagues [14]. It is now clear that the predominant somatostatin receptor subtype on most neuroendocrine tumors is subtype 2 [13,14].

The seminal work of Lamberts, Krenning, and Reubi and colleagues has led to the ability to radiolabel a modified octreotide analogue, tyrosine (Tyr)-3-octreotide, with iodine-123 (^{123}I) for in vivo, whole-body scintigraphy as well as iodine-125 (^{125}I) for in vitro autoradiography. This group first reported the diagnostic efficacy of ^{123}I-labeled (Tyr)-3-octreotide scintigraphy for both somatostatin-receptor-positive carcinoid and neuroendocrine tumors [16]. They reported visualizing carcinoid tumors in 12 of 13 patients (92%) and 7 of 9 patients (78%) with pancreatic neuroendocrine tumors. They also noted that symptomatic patients in whom neuroendocrine tumors were visualized did respond to octreotide therapy. O'Connor and colleagues [17] determined dosimetry and biodistribution of the ^{123}I-labeled somatostatin analogue (modified tyrosinated octreotide) in patients with neuroendocrine tumors. In their studies, neuroendocrine tumors were identified in 25 of 28 patients (89%). These studies demonstrated increased uptake and delayed clearance in liver, gallbladder, and intestine with less accumulation of label in the kidney and bladder. Their work suggested that the ^{123}I-labeled analogue may not be suitable for somatostatin-receptor-positive neuroendocrine tumors metastatic to the liver [17]. The Ohio State University Medical Center has had a large experience using the ^{123}I-tyrosinated somatostatin analogue as well [18]. Although several problems existed in using the ^{123}I label—particularly, the short half-life of ^{123}I, and also inconsistent labeling techniques from one scan to another—we were able to confirm the studies of both the Rotterdam [16] and Mayo Clinic [17] groups. Specifically, we were able to localize somatostatin-receptor-positive carcinoid tumors and such neuroendocrine tumors as gastrinoma, glucagonoma, and the childhood neuroendocrine tumor, neuroblastoma. We further determined that high-pressure liquid chromatography purification was not necessary in the preparation of the ^{123}-I somatostatin analogue labeling, and that a one-step SEP-PAK (Water Association, Milford, MA) column was adequate before scintigraphy. We further observed that the type and number of the tumor's somatostatin receptors were as important in obtaining visualization as the overall amount of the radiolabeled peptide used [18].

Commercial development of Octreoscan

The Rotterdam group, in collaboration with Mallinckrodt (Petten) and Sandoz (Basel), developed a very stable, easy-to-formulate indium-labeled octreotide compound referred to as *OctreoScan*. Figure 8-2 depicts the structure of the indium-111 pentetreotide structure. Pentetreotide is formed by conjugating the chelating agent diethylenetriaminepenta-acetic acid (DTPA) to octreotide. As can be noted, when comparing this structure with Figure 8-1 the amino acid residue and ringed structure are again maintained. Krenning and colleagues [19] have recently compiled their large clinical experience using both the ^{123}I-(Tyr)3 octreotide and indium-111 pentetreotide scintigraphy, and have correlated it with ^{125}I-(Tyr)3 octreotide autoradiography [19]. In addition to demonstrating the high correlation between radiolabeled somatostatin analogues and in vitro tumor somatostatin receptor positivity, the authors have also noted that granulomas and autoimmune processes can be visualized because of local accumulation of somatostatin-receptor-positive activated mononuclear leukocytes. They further note that in "many instances" a positive radiolabeled somatostatin scintigraphy predicts a favorable response to octreotide. A summary of octreotide dosage ranges for various neuroendocrine tumors in correlation with either scintigraphy or autoradiography is shown in Table 8-3 [20].

The figures in this chapter depict various Octreoscan scintigraphic–positive neuroendocrine tumors with conventional scintigraphy and scans and caveats from our Ohio State University Medical Center experience.

TABLE 8-1. EFFECTS OF SOMATOSTATIN

System	Effect	Product or Function Affected
Anterior pituitary		
Endocrine	Inhibited secretion	Growth hormone
		Thyrotropin (TSH)
Gastrointestinal tract		
Endocrine	Inhibited gut hormone secretion	Gastrin
		VIP
		Motilin
		Neurotensin
		GIP
Exocrine	Inhibited secretion	Acid
		Pepsin
		Fluid/electrolytes
Absorption	Inhibited absorption	Calcium
		Glucose
		Amino acids
		Triglycerides
Motility	Inhibition	Gastric emptying
		Small-bowel transit time
Mucosal protection	Cytoprotection	Stomach
		Duodenum
Hemodynamics	Decreased blood flow	Mesenteric and celiac arteries
Pancreas		
Endocrine	Inhibited secretion	Insulin
		Glucagon
		Pancreatic polypeptide
Exocrine	Inhibited secretion	Digestive enzymes
		Bicarbonate
Liver		
Hemodynamics	Decreased blood flow	Portal vein
Exocrine	Inhibited secretion	Bile acid–independent bile flow
Kidney		
Homeostasis	Balanced fluid and electrolytes	Diuresis

TABLE 8-1.

Effects of somatostatin. GIP—glucose-dependent insulinotropic peptide; VIP—vasoactive intestinal peptide. (*Adapted from* O'Dorisio and O'Dorisio [21]; with permission.)

TABLE 8-2. SOMATOSTATIN ANALOGUE'S RECEPTOR BINDING AND CLINICAL AND THERAPEUTIC CORRELATIONS

Tumor	Sign or symptom	Mean daily dose	Clinical response (1–10)	Comments
Growth hormone-producing	Acromegaly	215–670 µg	10	Headache, arthritic pain alleviated 80% scintigraphy (+) 100% somatostatin receptor (+)
Thyrotropin-producing	Hyperthyroidism and thyrotoxicosis	260–620 µg	9, biochemical 6, clinical	Considered agent of choice 2 of 2 scintigraphy (+) 2 of 2 somatostatin receptor (+)
Gastrinoma	Zollinger-Ellison syndrome	220–675 µg	6	Diarrhea, abdominal pain improved High dose may be needed 80%–100% scintigraphy (+) 100% somatostatin receptor (+)
Carcinoid	Carcinoid syndrome Flushing and diarrhea	450–1,350 µg three times	9.5	Flushing most responsive, also wheezing, when present 90%–98% scintigraphy (+) 80%–87% somatostatin receptor (+)
VIPoma	Watery diarrhea syndrome	250 µg	8	Effective in controlling secretory diarrhea 87% somatostatin receptor (+)
Glucagonoma	Glucagonoma syndrome	200–300 µg	8, rash 10, diarrhea	Rash responds over time Diarrhea responds Diabetes mellitus improves half the time Scintigraphy and receptor (+) in 3 of 3 patients
Insulinoma	Hypoglycemia	200–675 µg	4.5	Must watch for worsening of hypoglycemia 50% scintigraphy (+) 40% to 78% somatostatin receptor (+)
GHRFoma	Acromegaly	200–600 µg	8	Few reported cases Soft-tissue changes improve 100% scintigraphy (+) in 4 of 4 patients
PPoma	Asymptomatic or diarrhea (rare)	250–320 µg	10	Diarrhea, when present, resolves Few reported cases

TABLE 8-2.

Somatostatin analogue's receptor binding and clinical and therapeutic correlations. (*Adapted from* O'Dorisio and O'Dorisio [20]; with permission.)

TABLE 8-3. EFFECTS OF OCTREOTIDE

System	Effect	Potential Clinical Application
Gastrointestinal tract	↓ gastrointestinal hormone secretion	Endocrine tumors (carcinoid syndrome and VIPoma)*
	↓ intestinal fluid and electrolyte secretion	Secretory diarrhea (related to diabetes, AIDS, partial small-bowel obstruction, chemotherapy)
	↓ gastric acid/pepsin	Peptic ulcer
	↑ mucosal protection	
	↓ splanchnic blood flow	Upper gastrointestinal bleeding (variceal bleeding)
	↓ motility (gastric emptying)	Dumping syndrome, diarrhea
	↑ motility (low doses)	Scleroderma, pseudo-obstruction
Anterior pituitary gland	↓ growth hormone secretion	Acromegaly,* nonfunctional tumors, psoriasis, diabetic retinopathy
	↓ thyrotropin (TSH) secretion (chronic high doses)	TSHomas
Pancreas	↓ exocrine secretion	Pancreatitis, pseudocyst, pancreatic fistula
	↓ endocrine secretion	Endocrine tumors (gastrinoma, VIPoma)
Nervous system	↓ substance P release	Pain states (migraine headaches)
Solid tumors	Binds to somatostatin receptors	Breast, colorectal, ovarian, kidney, gastric, small-cell lung, pancreatic, lymphoma, or prostatic cancer
	↓ tumor growth (via epidermal growth factor, fibroblast growth factor, or insulin-like growth factor-1 levels)	
	↓ angiogenesis	

*Approved for clinical disease states in the United States.

TABLE 8-3.

Effects of octreotide. (*Adapted from* O'Dorisio and O'Dorisio [21]; with permission.)

TABLE 8-4. PEPTIDE AND PEPTIDE ANALOGUES: POTENTIAL CLINICAL APPLICATIONS

Peptide	Tumor	Application
Somatostatin	Carcinoid, neuroblastoma, gastrinoma	Imaging, radioreceptor-guided surgery
Substance P	Primitive neuro-ectodermal tumor, small-cell lung cancer	Antiproliferative Antagonist
Gastrin-releasing peptide	Colon, breast, small-cell lung cancer	Antiproliferative Antagonist
Epidermal growth factor	Melanoma, breast neuroblastoma, glioma	Antagonist
Insulin-like growth factor-1	Pancreatic, neuroblastoma, breast	Antagonist
Vasoactive intestinal peptide	Neuroblastoma, colon	Imaging, therapy
Neuropeptide Y	Neuroblastoma, primitive neuro-ectodermal tumor, pheochromocytoma	Diagnostic
Tumor necrosis factor-α	Colon, astrocytoma	Cytotoxicity
Luteinizing hormone-releasing hormone	Pituitary	Antagonist

TABLE 8-4.

Peptide and peptide analogues: potential clinical applications. (*Adapted from* O'Dorisio and O'Dorisio [21]; with permission.)

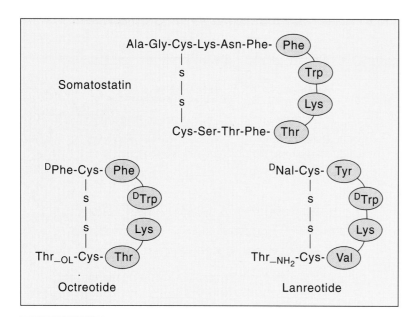

FIGURE 8-1.

The amino acid residue structure of somatostatin and two congeners are shown. The Trp-Lys residues are retained in both synthetic compounds, and appear to be of primary importance as the somatostatin and its congeners' binding unit. (*Adapted from* O'Dorisio *et al.* [22]; with permission.)

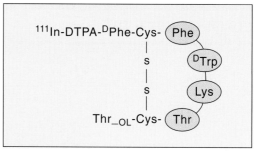

FIGURE 8-2.

Pentetreotide is formed by conjugating the chelating agent DTPA to octreotide, enabling radiolabeling with indium 111 (^{111}In). The two amino acid residues try-lys are again retained (*see* Figure 8-1) in the ^{111}In-labeled analogue. This compound is commercially marketed as Octreoscan (Mallinckrodt [Petten] and Sandoz [Basel]). (*Adapted from* O'Dorisio *et al.* [22]; with permission.)

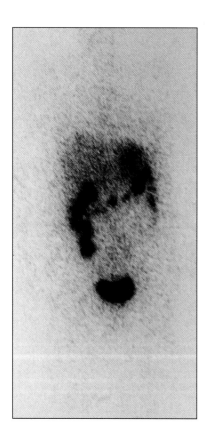

FIGURE 8-3.

Iodine-123-tyrosine-3-octreotide anterior whole-body scintigraph demonstrates extensive physiologic gastrointestinal (GI) activity that interferes with interpretation of the abdomen as regards sites of possible pathology.

This radiopharmaceutical is excreted primarily through the GI tract and represented one of the early attempts to develop a clinically useful somatostatin analogue for imaging purposes. The extensive GI excretion of this radiopharmaceutical severely limited its usefulness for evaluating patients suspected of gastroenteropancreatic neuroendocrine tumors.

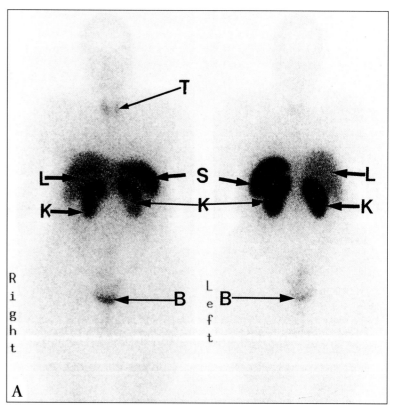

FIGURE 8-4.

Normal study. These Indium (In)-111 pentetreotide whole-body scintigraphs demonstrate sites of normally increased activity. **A,** Thyroid, liver, spleen, kidney, and bladder activity, as well as slight gastrointestinal activity that has been reduced by the use of cathartics.

(*continued on next page*)

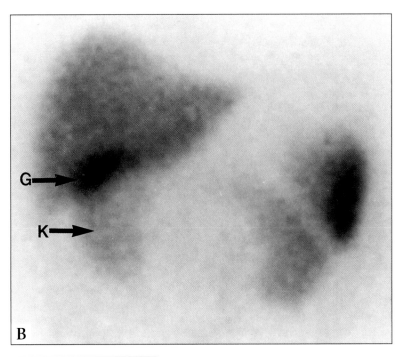

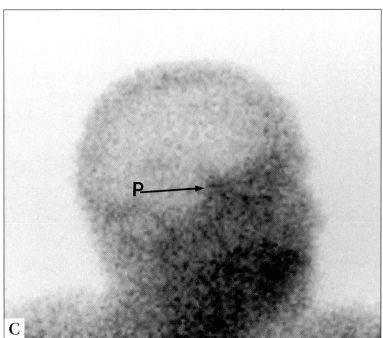

B

C

FIGURE 8-4. (CONTINUED)

B, Planar anterior scintigraph of the liver demonstrates normal gallbladder activity (seen more frequently with single photon emission computed tomography [SPECT] imaging). **C,** The anterior pituitary gland possesses somatostatin receptors and may also be visualized on planar and SPECT images of the head.

Approximately 2% of In-111 pentetreotide and its breakdown products undergo hepatoenteric excretion; the other 98% is cleared by the kidneys. This allows for easier evaluation of the abdomen; however, because of the extensive physiologic uptake of the radiopharmaceutical by organs in the upper abdomen, it is essential to perform SPECT imaging of this area if pathology is suspected. B—urinary bladder; G—gallbladder; K—kidney; L—liver; P—pancreas; S—spleen; T—thyroid.

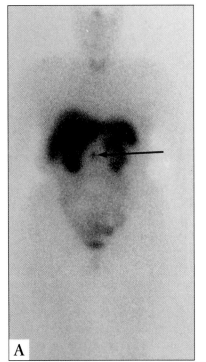

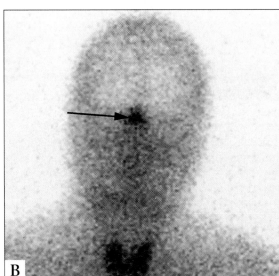

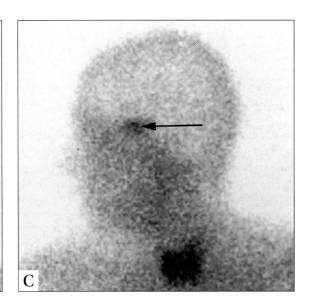

A

B

C

FIGURE 8-5.

This patient is a 46-year-old woman with multiple endocrine neoplasia-1 syndrome who previously underwent partial parathyroidectomy. **A,** Indium (In)-111 pentetreotide anterior whole-body scintigraphy revealed focal, abnormally increased activity (*arrow*) in the midline of the upper abdomen. Laparotomy showed this to be a gastrinoma in the body of the pancreas. Also noted on the anterior whole-body scintigraph is somewhat prominent activity in the anticipated location of the pituitary gland. **B–C,** Planar anterior and lateral views of the head demonstrated increased pituitary activity (*arrows*), which was also well delineated by single photon emission computed tomography imaging (**panels D** and **E**). Subsequent craniotomy and immunohistology revealed the pituitary lesion to be a 2-cm prolactinoma.

(*continued on next page*)

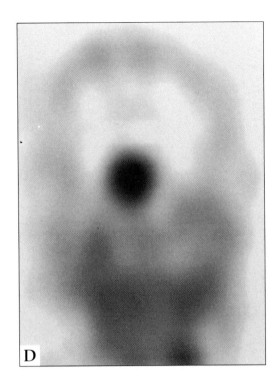

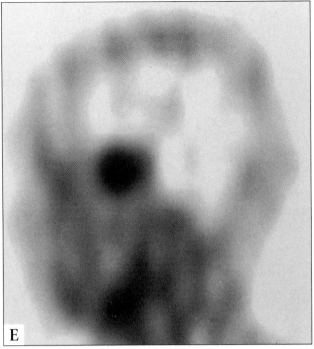

FIGURE 8-5. (CONTINUED)

Approximately 90% of gastrinomas are visualized by scintigraphy. Although MR imaging and computed tomography remain the preferred modalities for evaluation of the pituitary and hypothalamic region, a high percentage of hyperfunctioning thyroid-stimulating hormone-producing, growth hormone-producing, and prolactin-producing anterior pituitary adenomas are visualized by In-111 pentetreotide scintigraphy. Hyperfunctioning adrenocorticotropic hormone-producing anterior pituitary adenomas and posterior pituitary tumors are reportedly not visualized by In-111 pentetreotide scintigraphy.

D (left) **E** (right)

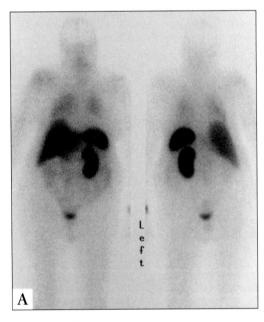

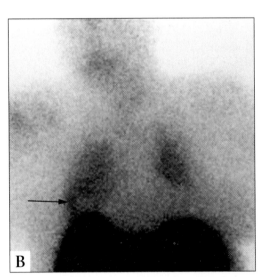

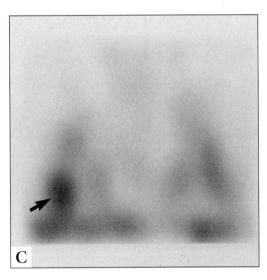

A **B** **C**

FIGURE 8-6.

A 74-year-old woman with a previous history of right-middle lobe lung resection for paraganglioma 21 years before and right nephrectomy for renal cell carcinoma 9 years before being admitted for evaluation of Cushing's syndrome. MR imaging of the head was normal. Dexamethasone suppression test was consistent with ectopic adrenocorticotropic hormone (ACTH) secretion. **A**, Indium (In)-111 whole-body scintigraphy demonstrated diffuse pulmonary activity that was believed to reflect chronic aspiration pneumonitis. **B**, An In-111 pentetreotide planar anterior scintigraph revealed a suspicious focal area of accentuated activity (*arrow*) laterally at the base of the right lung. **C–D**, Coronal single photon emission computed tomography images of the chest demonstrated a focal lesion (*arrows*) at the same location. Subsequent immunohistology proved this lesion to be a 9-mm ACTH-secreting carcinoid tumor.

Most ectopic ACTH-secreting tumors are bronchial carcinoid tumors. These tumors generally are well localized by In-111 pentetreotide scintigraphy whereas hyperfunctioning ACTH-secreting pituitary adenomas are rarely, if ever, visualized by In-111 pentetreotide scintigraphy. The diffuse pulmonary uptake seen in this case probably reflects influx of somatostatin receptor-bearing, activated lymphocytes into the lung parenchyma in response to chronic aspiration pneumonia. Positive In-111 pentetreotide scintigraphy in a number of other pulmonary diseases has also been reported. These include both small-cell and nonsmall-cell lung carcinoma, granulomatous diseases, and other inflammatory processes that are believed to be either associated with migration of activated lymphocytes into the area with or without proliferation of neuroendocrine cells that are normally found in the lung.

(*continued on next page*)

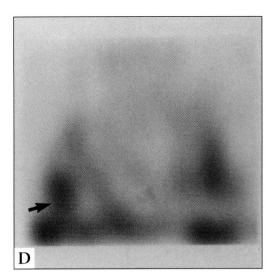

D

FIGURE 8-6. (CONTINUED)

Although whole-body scintigraphs are a handy screening method, planar "spot views" obtained for a minimum of 10 to 15 minutes are believed to be more sensitive for the detection of some of these small somatostatin receptor–positive tumors.

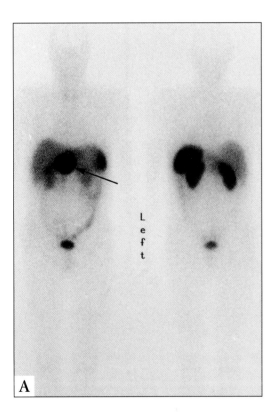

A

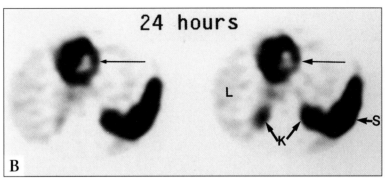

B

FIGURE 8-7.

A 58-year-old man with biopsy-proven carcinoid tumor involving the liver had indium (In)-111 pentetreotide scintigraphy for documentation of other possible sites of metastatic involvement. **A,** Whole-body scintigraphs demonstrated a prominent lesion (*arrow*) involving the junction of the right and the left hepatic lobes. **B,** Single photon emission computed tomography images in the transaxial plane revealed the tumor (*arrows*) to have a "cold" center that represented partial infarction of this tumor.

This tumor was large and was also easily demonstrated by ultrasonography. It is well recognized, however, that neuroendocrine tumors smaller than 1 cm may be seen by In-111 pentetreotide scintigraphy, and yet frequently will be undetected by conventional imaging modalities, such as computed tomography, MR imaging, and ultrasonography. L–liver; K–kidney; S–spleen.

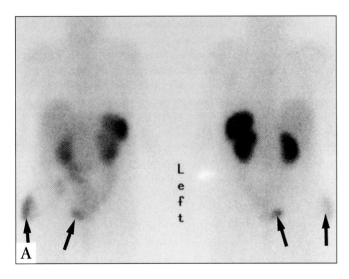

A

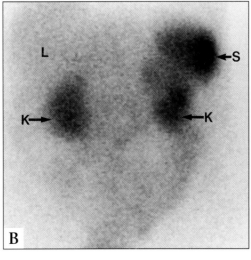

B

FIGURE 8-8.

A 65-year-old woman complaining of vague abdominal pain had undergone colonic resection for carcinoid tumor 5 months before this study. Indium-111 pentetreotide whole-body scintigraphs (**panel A**) and planar view of the upper abdomen (**panel B**) were unremarkable except for prominent gastrointestinal activity and contamination (*arrows*) involving the lateral aspect of the right hip and lower pelvic area.

(*continued on next page*)

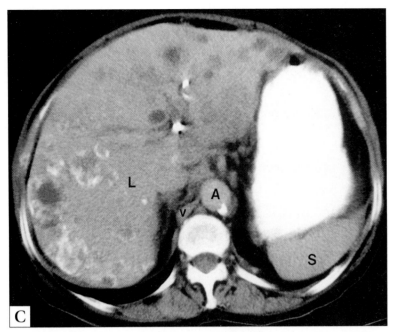

FIGURE 8-8. (*CONTINUED*)

Note the absence of any focal abnormalities involving the liver. C, Contrast-enhanced computed tomographic (CT) examination revealed extensive multiple large metastases involving the liver.

Some patients with focal hepatic metastases from carcinoid, medullary thyroid carcinoma, and small-cell lung carcinoma may have normal scintigraphs, even when the metastases are readily identified by other imaging modalities (*ie*, CT, ultrasonography, MR imaging). Explanation for this discrepancy is believed to relate to activity in the lesions that is similar to the physiologic uptake in the remainder of the liver. This may be reflecting a tumor with a relatively low density of somatostatin receptor or tumor with a subtype of somatostatin receptor that does not have a high affinity for octreotide. A—aorta; K—kidney; L—liver; S—spleen; V—vena cava.

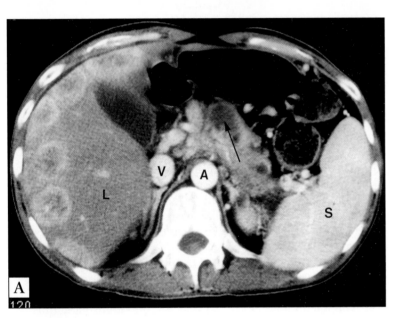

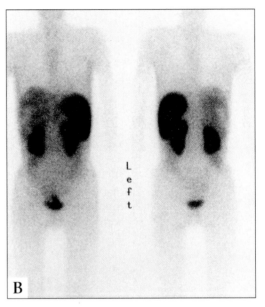

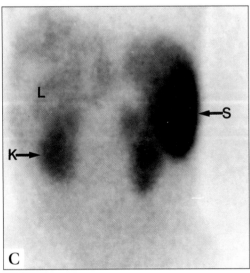

FIGURE 8-9.

A 25-year-old man was being evaluated for abdominal pain of 3 months' duration. A, Contrast-enhanced computed tomography of the abdomen demonstrated multiple hepatic lesions as well as a lesion in the head of the pancreas (*arrow*). A percutaneous liver biopsy was performed and suggested a diagnosis of "tumor wth neuroendocrine characteristics". Indium-111 pentetreotide whole-body scintigraphy (**panel B**) and anterior spot view of the upper abdomen (**panel C**) revealed multiple focal "cold" defects scattered throughout the liver. Subsequent debulking surgery was performed and revealed the tumor to be an adenocarcinoma of the pancreas with extensive metastatic involvement of the liver.

The absence of uptake of the radiopharmaceutical by the tumor and metastases suggests that it is a non-neuroendocrine tumor. It has been shown, however, that neuroendocrine tumors with very-low-affinity receptors for the radiopharmaceutical or a low density of receptors may fail to be visualized by scintigraphy, and that their metastases may present as cold hepatic defects. Neuroendocrine tumors that dedifferentiate to a more anaplastic form may also fail to be visualized. A—aorta; K—kidney; L—liver; S—spleen; V—vena cava.

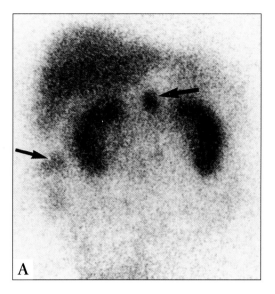

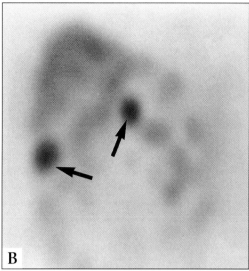

FIGURE 8-10.

This 64-year-old woman complained of diarrhea and glucose intolerance. She had a history of malignant glucagonoma, for which she underwent surgical resection (Whipple's procedure) 5 years previously, plus excision of recurrent tumor approximately 14 months before the study shown. Planar view of the upper abdomen (**panel A**) and single photon emission computed tomography (SPECT) image in the coronal plane (**panel B**) identified lesions (*arrows*) in the midline and caudal to the right hepatic lobe. Exploratory laparotomy using radiation-guided surgery revealed metastatic glucagonoma at these sites.

Most islet cell tumors are well demonstrated by indium-111 pentetreotide scintigraphy. SPECT imaging of the upper abdomen, however, is required for better evaluation of the pancreatic area because of interfering hepatic, renal, splenic, and occasionally gastrointestinal activity on the planar images.

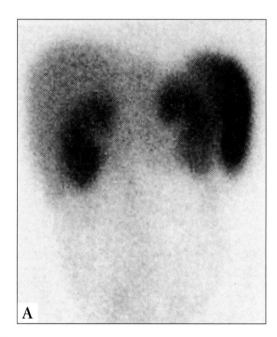

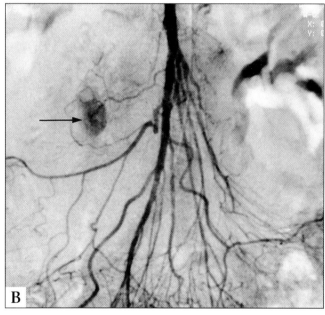

FIGURE 8-11.

A 75-year-old woman who was admitted to the hospital for the evaluation of syncope and mental status changes was noted to have inappropriately elevated levels of plasma insulin. **A**, An Indium (In)-111 pentetreotide planar anterior view and single photon emission computed tomography images of the upper abdomen were normal. Computed tomography image of the upper abdomen did not reveal any abnormality involving the pancreas. **B**, Angiography demonstrated a hypervascular focus (*arrow*) in the head of the pancreas. The lesion was enucleated at surgery and proved to be a 1.3 cm insulinoma by immunohistology.

Approximately 50% of patients with insulinoma will have normal results with In-111 pentetreotide scintigraphy. These insulinomas may express a subtype of somatostatin receptor that does not concentrate the radiopharmaceutical adequately for imaging purposes. It is also possible that some insulinomas may have either no receptors or may have an inadequate number of receptors to allow for their detection by scintigraphy.

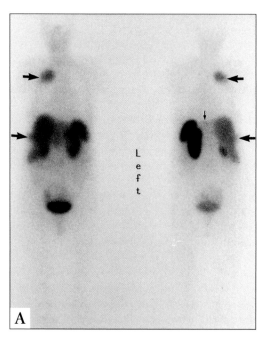 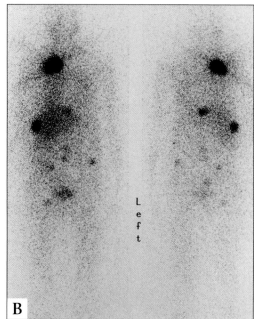

Figure 8-12.

This 78-year-old woman underwent resection of a right adrenal pheochromocytoma and right nephrectomy 20 years previously. She was brought to the emergency department for a syncopal episode, at which time she was noted to be hypertensive. A chest radiograph revealed a 6-cm right upper lobe mass. Endocrine profile suggested possible metastatic pheochromocytoma. **A,** Indium (In)-111 pentetreotide whole-body scintigraphs identified the right upper lobe lesion, an abnormality lateral to the right lobe of the liver, and a suspicious area in the lower thoracic spine (*arrows*). **B,** I-131 metaiodobenzylguanidine (MIBG) whole-body scintigraphs revealed additional lesions scattered throughout the abdomen and in the right groin, plus they provided better delineation of the lower thoracic spine lesions and the lesion lateral to the right hepatic lobe.

Studies have indicated that both MIBG and pentetreotide are each approximately 90% sensitive for the identification of pheochromocytoma. As in this case, the two radiopharmaceuticals may not always identify the same lesions. Some authors prefer MIBG over pentetreotide because of less interference from renal activity in the region of the adrenal glands. In-111 pentetreotide scintigraphy, on the other hand, has been proposed as a method for predicting tumor responsiveness to octreotide therapy in metastatic pheochromocytoma, as well as in other neuroendocrine tumors.

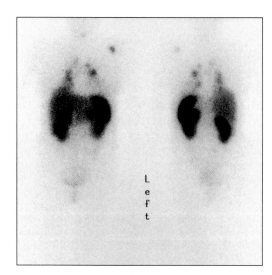

Figure 8-13.

This 40-year-old woman with a history of prior thyroidectomy for medullary thyroid carcinoma (MTC) was being evaluated for rising serum calcitonin levels. Indium (In)-111 pentetreotide anterior and posterior whole-body scintigraphs reveal multiple focal areas of abnormally increased activity involving the chest, region of the left shoulder, skull, and neck.

MTC is one of the neuroendocrine tumors that may express various subtypes of somatostatin receptors, some of which have little, if any, affinity for In-111 pentetreotide. Approximately one half to two thirds of patients with metastatic MTC are reported to have abnormal scintigraphic results. Carcinoembryonic antigen (CEA) is an independent marker for dedifferentiation of MTC. MTC dedifferentiation, as may be reflected by a fall in the calcitonin to CEA ratio, also may be associated with normal scintigraphs in the presence of metastatic MTC.

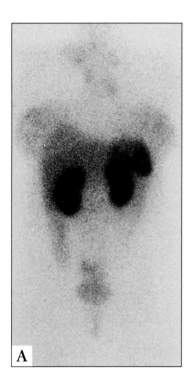

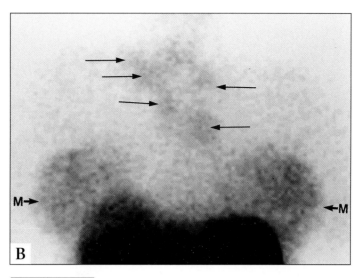

B

demonstrate abnormal moderately increased activity in the supraclavicular regions, mediastinum, and perihilar areas (*arrows*), which represents active disease. Increased breast activity associated with lactation is also identified.

The role of In-111 pentetreotide scintigraphy for the evaluation of lymphomas remains under investigation. Preliminary data suggest that In-111 pentetreotide scintigraphy may not prove to be as efficacious as was hoped in the staging of lymphomas, but may have a role in predicting the responsiveness of this and other diseases to therapy with octreotide. M—mammary gland.

FIGURE 8-14.

This 28-year-old woman with known Hodgkin's disease was 6 months postpartum and still nursing up to the time of this study. Indium (In)-111 pentetreotide anterior whole-body scintigraph (**panel A**) and planar image of the chest (**panel B**)

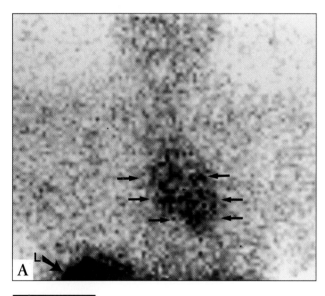

A

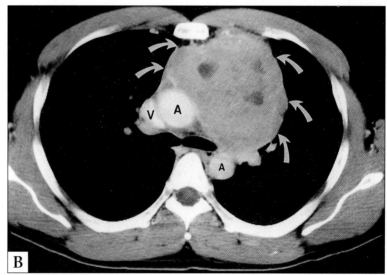

B

FIGURE 8-15.

This 31-year-old man with non-Hodgkin's lymphoma had indium-111 pentetreotide scintigraphy performed, including a planar anterior view of the chest (**panel A**), which demonstrated abnormal moderately increased mediastinal activity (*arrows*). **B**, Contrast-enhanced computed tomography examination of the chest revealed a large mediastinal mass (*arrows*). The patient underwent fiberoptic bronchoscopy and left anterior mediastinotomy

with biopsy that confirmed the mass to be non-Hodgkin's lymphoma.

Preliminary data indicate that non-Hodgkin's lymphoma is less likely to be detected than Hodgkin's disease. Interestingly, unlike most other neuroendocrine tumors, the less differentiated tumors in the non-Hodgkin's group are reported to be detected more frequently than those which are better differentiated. A—aorta; L—lymphoma; V—vena cava.

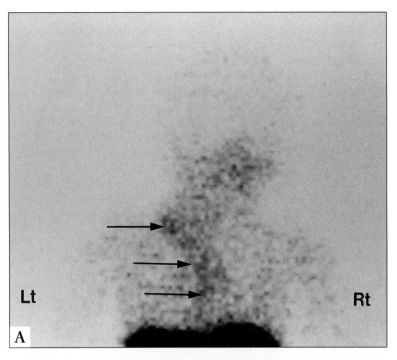

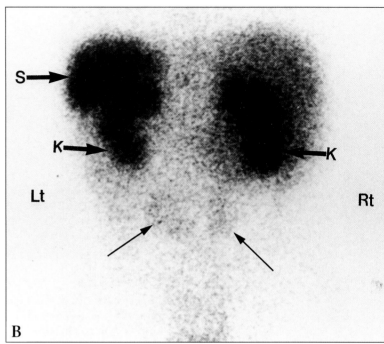

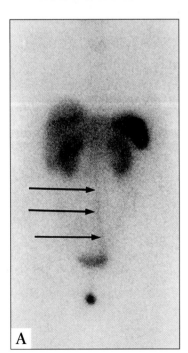

FIGURE 8-16.

This 5-year-old boy with neuroblastoma underwent indium (In)-111 pentetreotide scintigraphy. **A–B,** Planar posterior views of the head and trunk revealed abnormal focally increased activity at the left supraclavicular region, paraspinal region, and in the lower abdomen (*arrows*). **C,** Contrast-enhanced computed tomography of the abdomen demonstrated a large retroperitoneal mass (*arrows*) encircling the aorta. Surgical pathology reported metastatic neuroblastoma.

In-111 pentetreotide has been reported to be as equally effective as radioiodinated metaiodobenzylguanidine (MIBG) in localizing both primary and metastatic neuroblastoma. Intensive renal accumulation of In-111 pentetreotide versus radioiodinated MIBG continues to make MIBG the preferred agent for evaluating these patients in many pediatric nuclear medicine departments. A—aorta; K—kidney; S—spleen.

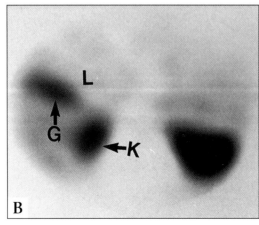

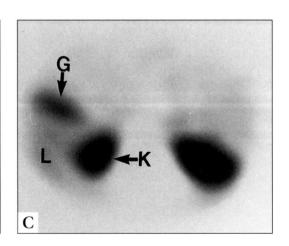

FIGURE 8-17.

Normal variants and other entities may result in accumulation of Indium-111 pentetreotide. **A,** An uncomplicated abdominal surgical scar (*arrows*) in this patient who underwent abdominal laparotomy 8 weeks before the study was done. **B–C,** The gallbladder is demonstrated on these transaxial single photon emission computed tomography (SPECT) images of the liver. Because of its location and shape, it should not be mistaken for a lesion.

(*continued on next page*)

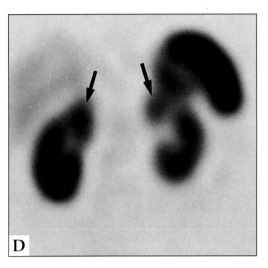 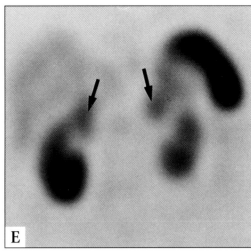 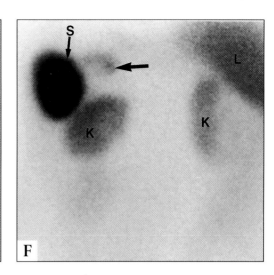

FIGURE 8-17. (CONTINUED)

D–E, Fetal lobulation of the kidney on SPECT examination of the upper abdomen may at times mimic an adrenal mass (*arrow*) on some coronal images. F, Splenosis or accessory splenic tissue (*arrow*) may also cause difficulty in evaluating the upper abdomen in patients suspected of neuroendocrine tumors. G—gallbladder; K—kidney; L—liver; S—spleen.

REFERENCES

1. Bayliss WM, Starling EH: The mechanism of pancreatic secretion. *J Physiol (Lond)* 1902, 28:325–353.

2. Redfern J, O'Dorisio TM: Gastrointestinal hormones and carcinoid syndrome. In *Endocrinology and Metabolism*, edn 3. Edited by Felig P, Baxter JD, Frohman LA. New York: McGraw-Hill, Inc; 1995:1675–1702.

3. Walsh JH: Gastrointestinal peptide hormones. In *Gastrointestinal Disease: Pathophysiology, Diagnosis, Management*, edn 4. Edited by Sleisenger MH, Fordtran JS. Philadelphia: WB Saunders; 1989:78–107.

4. Brazeau P, Vale W, Burgus R, *et al.*: Hypothalamic polypeptide that inhibits the secretion of immunoreactive pituitary growth hormone. *Science* 1972, 179:77–79.

5. O'Dorisio TM, Redfern JS: Somatostatin and somatostatin-like peptides: Clinical research and clinical applications. In *Advances in Endrocrinology and Metabolism*. Edited by Mazzaferri EL. Chicago: Mosby-Year Book; 1990:185–230.

6. Reichlin S: Somatostatin: Historical aspects. *Scand J Gastroenterol* 1986, 21:1–10.

7. Bauer W, Briner U, Doepfner W, *et al.*: A very potent and selective octapeptide analog of somatostatin with prolonged action. *Life Sci* 1982, 31:1133–1140.

8. Redfern JS, O'Dorisio TM: Therapeutic uses of gastrointestinal peptides. *Endocrinol Metab Clin North Am* 1993, 22:845–873.

9. Harris AG, O'Dorisio TM, Woltering EA, *et al.*: Consensus statement: Octreotide dose titration in secretory diarrhea. *Dig Dis Sci* 1995, 40:1464–1473.

10. Chen F, O'Dorisio MS, Hermann GE, *et al.*: Mechanisms of action of long-acting analogs of somatostatin. *Regul Pept* 1993, 44:285–295.

11. Hsu WH, Xiang H, Rajan AS, *et al.*: Somatostatin inhibits insulin secretion by a G-protein mediated decrease in Ca^{2+} entry through voltage-dependent Ca^{2+} channels in beta cells. *J Biol Chem* 1991, 266:837–843.

12. Liebow C, Lee MT, Schally A: Antitumor effects of somatostatin mediated by the stimulation of tyrosine phosphatase. *Metabolism* 1990, 39:163–166.

13. Woltering EA, O'Dorisio MS, O'Dorisio TM: The role of radiolabelled somatostatin analogues in the management of cancer patients. In *Principles and Progress in Oncology: Updates*. Edited by DeVita VT, Hellman S, Rosenberg SA. Philadelphia: JB Lippincott; 1995:9:1–15.

14. Reubi JC, Hacki WH, Lamberts SWJ: Hormone-producing gastrointestinal tumors contain a high density of somatostatin receptors. *J Clin Endocrinol Metab* 1987, 65:1127–1134.

15. Lamberts SWJ, Hofland LJ, von Koetsveld PM, *et al.*: Parallel in vivo and in vitro detection of functional somatostatin receptors in human endocrine pancreatic tumors: Consequences with regard to diagnosis, localization and therapy. *J Clin Endocrinol Metab* 1990, 71:566–574.

16. Lamberts SWJ, Bakker WH, Reubi J-C, Krenning EP: Somatostatin-receptor imaging in the localization of endocrine tumors. *N Engl J Med* 1990, 323:1246–1249.

17. O'Connor MK, Kvols LK, Brown ML, *et al.*: Dosimetry and biodistribution of an iodine-123-labeled somatostatin analog in patients with neuroendocrine tumors. *J Nucl Med* 1992, 33:1613–1619.

18. Schirmer TP, O'Dorisio TM, Olsen JO, *et al.*: Influence of isotope dose on somatostatin receptor imaging: When less is better. *Semin Oncol* 1994, 21(suppl):51–55.

19. Krenning EP, Kwekkeboom DJ, Bakker WH, *et al.*: Somatostatin receptor scintigraphy with [^{111}In-DTPA-D-Phe^1]- and [^{123}I-TYR^3]-octreotide: The Rotterdam experience with more than 1,000 patients. *Eur J Nucl Med* 1993, 20:716–731.

20. O'Dorisio TM, O'Dorisio MS: Neural crest tumors: Rationale for somatostatin and its analogs in diagnosis and therapy. In *Endocrine Tumors*. Edited by Mazzaferri EL, Samaan NA. Boston: Blackwell Scientific; 1993:531–542.

21. O'Dorisio TM, O'Dorisio MS: Clinical and therapeutic implications of gastrointestinal peptides and their analogs. *New Perspectives in Cancer Diagnosis and Management* 1995, 3:41–46.

22. O'Dorisio TM, O'Dorisio MS, Owyang C: Rational and clinical application of neuropeptide congeners for diagnosis and therapy of neuroendocrine tumors. *Regulatory Peptide Letter* 1994, 3:52–55.

Chapter 9

Cystic Fibrosis

P E T E R   R .   D U R I E

Cystic fibrosis (CF) is the most common lethal autosomal recessive disorder among whites. It is a generalized disease that affects various secreting epithelial tissues, but clinical evidence is provided by pulmonary and gastrointestinal manifestations. Heterozygotes with one normal CF allele and one mutant allele are entirely asymptomatic. A child born to two CF carriers has a one-in-four chance of being affected with CF by acquiring a mutation from each parent. Disease frequency varies considerably among ethnic groups; it is highest among people of Northern European origin, among whom approximately 1 in 2500 births is affected. It is extremely rare in people of Asian or African origin.

Despite considerable advances in clinical ability to identify specific CF mutations, the diagnosis of CF is still established by quantitative sweat iontophoresis. This test is based on the observation by di Sant'Agnese and colleagues that the concentration of salt in the sweat of CF patients is greatly elevated [1]. In the 1930s, it was separated from other celiac syndromes by identifying the dual involvement of the pancreas and the lungs in affected patients [2,3]. At that time, the demonstration of pancreatic insufficiency was the key to the clinical diagnosis. In the 1950s, Gibbs, Bostick, and Smith [4] showed that steatorrhea was not seen in all patients. Since then, it has become increasingly apparent that the clinical expression of the disease is extremely variable.

In the years before the CF gene was identified, research into the etiopathogenesis of this disorder was hampered by the inability to differentiate the basic defect from secondary effects of the disease. Most research strategies were based on identifying differences between heterozygotes and affected individuals in cells and bodily fluids. Over a period of more than 4 decades of research, no protein or biochemical abnormality was identified that could be convincingly viewed as the primary defect. In contrast, electrophysiologic studies were quite helpful. Quinton initially showed that chloride permeation was defective in the sweat duct [5]; this work was quickly followed by evidence of a similar defect in the respiratory tract epithelium. Subsequent work in the isolated secretory coil of the sweat gland, respiratory epithelium [6], and isolated secretory cells in culture demonstrated that affected epithelia had unresponsive cyclic AMP (cAMP)–mediated chloride channels within the apical membrane [7]. These observations were confirmed after the CF gene was cloned [8]. Patch clamp techniques have been used to show that specific chloride channels that open in the presence of cAMP–dependent protein kinase and ATP in normal cells do not do so in cells cultured from CF patients [9].

The predominant clinical feature of CF is respiratory tract involvement, in which obstruction of airways by sticky mucus gives rise to infection, especially with *pseudomonas* species. Most patients experience gastrointestinal difficulties; 85% show pancreatic insufficiency caused by obstruction of small pancreatic ducts. Among neonates, over 10% of affected patients present with bowel obstruction resulting from meconium ileus. Up to 5% of patients develop overt liver disease, frequently in adolescence or adulthood [10]. Subclinical liver

disease is much more common, however. Infertility among affected males is virtually universal. Undernutrition is a cause of morbidity in affected children, adolescents, and young adults [11].

In most patients, the prognosis depends entirely on the pulmonary complications. Symptoms of airway disease usually begin insidiously as chronic pulmonary infection caused by the plugging of small airways by thick viscid secretion, which in turn leads to widespread destruction of the bronchioles, bronchiectasis, atelectasis, and emphysema with progressive respiratory failure and death. Over the past 2 to 3 decades, however, considerable improvement has been made in survival rates throughout the world. Median survival for patients in Canada is 32 years for males and 28 years for females. The great discrepancy in survival between sexes remains unexplained. Females appear to do almost as well as males until the early teens, but in late adolescence and adulthood deteriorate at a much faster rate [12]. Both males and females who do not have sufficient pancreatic disease to produce steatorrhea have better pulmonary function than their more common counterparts with pancreatic insufficiency [13].

■ GENETIC AND ELECTROPHYSIOLOGIC BASIS OF CYSTIC FIBROSIS

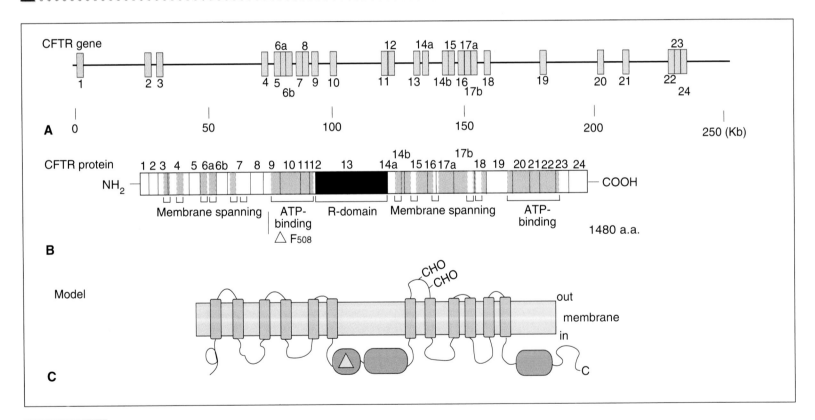

FIGURE 9-1.

A–C, Identification of the cystic fibrosis (CF) gene. In 1989, following concerted efforts by various investigators throughout the world, the CF gene was identified by Lap-Chee Tsui and J. Riordan of the University of Toronto, in collaboration with Francis Collins of the University of Michigan [8]. The CF gene, which is on the long arm of chromosome 7, comprises 27 exons spanning 230 kb of DNA. The gene product (initially thought to be comprised of 24 exons), named

the *cystic fibrosis transmembrane conductance regulator* (CFTR), is a protein of 1480 amino acids. The predominant mutation, which accounts for approximately 70% of all the CFTR gene mutations worldwide, is a three base-pair deletion in exon 10 of the CFTR gene, which results in the loss of a single amino acid, phenylalanine, at codon 508 (ΔF508). (*Adapted from* Tsui [14].)

FIGURE 9-2.

The deduced primary amino acid sequence of the cystic fibrosis transmembrane conductance regulator (CFTR) immediately suggested that the gene product was a membrane channel. This schematic model of the CFTR protein, which is situated within the cell membrane, shows membrane-spanning helices on each half of the molecule, which is shown as cylinders. The green spheres show two nucleotide binding folds (NBF); the light blue sphere shows large polar regulatory domain (R domain). Individual charged amino acids within the R domain are shown. Potential phosphorylation sites and N-glycosylation linkages are as shown. The predicted amino acid sequence of CFTR showed striking homology to a superfamily of membrane-associated proteins involved in active transport known as the ATP-binding cassette (ABC) superfamily. Members of this superfamily have several features in common, notably the presence of transmembrane domains and nucleotide binding folds. (*Adapted from* Riordan [8].)

NBF

R domain

Ψ N-linked carbohydrates

$\triangledown$ Protein Kinase C

$\blacktriangle$ Protein Kinase A

$\oplus$ Lysine, Arginine, and Histidine

$\ominus$ Aspartate and Glutamine

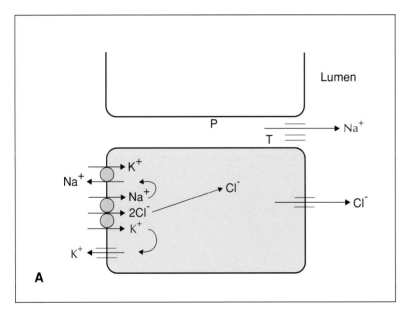

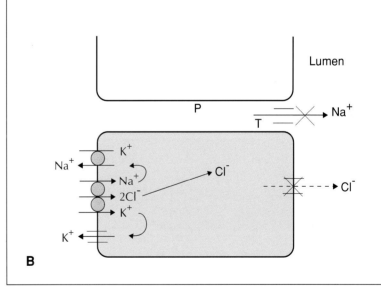

FIGURE 9-3.

Epithelial cell transport. **A,** Apical chloride channels are important elements in the secretion of sodium chloride by epithelial cells. In a typical epithelial cell, basolateral membrane transport processes give rise to accumulation of chloride intracellularly to levels that exceed the electrochemical potential in the cell exterior. When the apical chloride channel opens, the electrochemical gradient allows chloride to exit through the apical membrane. This generates a lumen-negative voltage that stimulates exit of sodium through paracellular-tight junctions. Secretion of water follows the movement of sodium and chloride. **B,** In cystic fibrosis, the cystic fibrosis transmembrane conductance regulator chloride channel is absent or defective. Consequently, chloride efflux from the apical membrane is impaired, which in turn prevents the movements of sodium paracellularly. The net *effect* of defective apical chloride channels would lead to diminished secretory volume. Na^+—sodium; Cl^-—chloride; K^+—potassium; P—paracellular route; T—tight junction. The *circles* in the basolateral membrane denote coupled ion transporters. (*Adapted from* Forstner and Durie [15].)

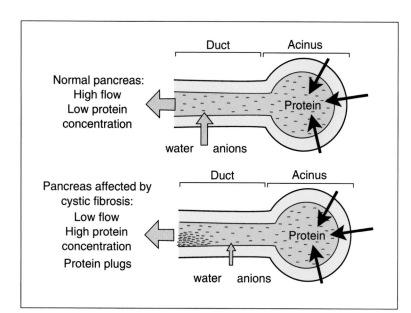

FIGURE 9-4.

The pancreas affected by cystic fibrosis is most vulnerable to lumenal concentration defects caused by the high protein content of acinar secretions and dependence on ductal cystic fibrosis transmembrane conductance regulator for anion (chloride and bicarbonate) and fluid secretion. When ductal water flow is reduced owing to defective anion secretion, protein concentration in the duct rises. High protein concentration causes precipitation of protein and plugging of duct lumina [16,17]. In contrast, the sweat duct is unaffected pathologically because of low protein load and high flow rate. (*Adapted from* Forstner and Durie [15].)

PATHOLOGY

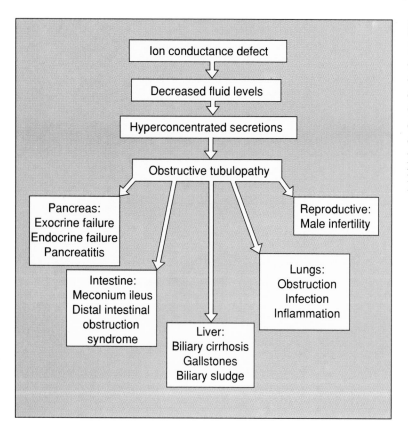

FIGURE 9-5.

Pathophysiology of cystic fibrosis. The ion conductance defect in epithelial tissues almost always results in reduced fluid flow within epithelia of organs normally possessing cystic fibrosis transmembrane conductance regulator (CFTR) expression. Absent or dysfunctional CFTR would be expected to lead to functional consequences in organs with a high concentration of macromolecules in the lumen of the ducts. A variety of organs listed in this figure are affected pathologically when proteins or other macromolecules precipitate, form plugs, slow ductal flow, and lead to blockage. (*Adapted from* Forstner and Durie [15].)

TABLE 9-1. THE PATHOLOGY OF CYSTIC FIBROSIS

ORGAN	PHYSIOLOGIC CHANGES	PATHOLOGY
Lung	Distal airway obstruction, glandular hyperplasia, mucous hypersecretion	Early—terminal bronchiolar plugging, peribronchiolar inflammation Late—mucus casts, atelectasis, bronchiectasis, emphysema, cor pulmonale
Pancreas	Decreased volume and increased concentration of secretions	Early—duct plugging, dilatation, acinar atrophy Late—fibrous and fatty replacement, and loss of islets
Intestine	Concentrated secretions, mucus altered—hyperglycosylated and hypersulfated	Meconium plug, distal ileum; crypt dilatation; meconium peritonitis; distal intestinal obstruction syndrome; constipation
Liver	Reduced bile salt secretion, increased circulating bile salt concentration	Early—bile ductular hyperplasia, eosinophilic plugging of intrahepatic bile duct, focal biliary cirrhosis Late—multilobular cirrhosis
Gallbladder	Reduced bile salt pool, lithogenic bile	Cystic duct occlusion, hypoplastic gallbladder, gallstones
Salivary glands	High calcium concentration	Inspissated mucus in intercalated ducts, mild inflammation
Epididymis and vas deferens	Reduced secretions	Absent—fibrous replacement

TABLE 9-1.

Pathology of cystic fibrosis (CF). Nearly all lesions in the disease have an obstructive element whereby a duct or air passage is blocked by mucus and/or other proteins. The airway and pancreatic lesions have the most adverse effects on health, but hepatic, intestinal, and reproductive tissues are also significantly affected pathologically. The pathologic changes closely mirror CF transmembrane conductance regulator (CFTR) expression on the epithelial cell surface of the respective organs.

The lung is not affected until after birth. Mucous plugging of small bronchioles and local inflammation are the earliest features. There is impaired clearance of airway secretions, which allows chronic infections to develop in the small airways, giving rise to chronic inflammation and progressive damage.

In contrast to the lung, the pancreas is affected in utero. At birth, intralobar ducts are plugged with proteinaceous material. Acinar cells show progressive atrophy. In time, both acini and proximal ducts atrophy and are replaced by fibrous tissue and fat. In the early stages, endocrine elements are relatively preserved, but islets also begin to disappear during adolescence. CF-associated diabetes mellitus is a common problem among adolescents and adults.

The intestine may also be affected in utero because of the low flow rate of intestinal contents. Rubbery masses of meconium may accumulate and obstruct the terminal ileum, giving rise to meconium ileus. After birth, predominantly in adolescence and adulthood, intermittent subacute intestinal obstruction with inspissated mucofeculent material is common.

CF-associated liver disease is characterized by small biliary ducts obstructed by eosinophilic material. This produces a patchy form of liver disease, focal biliary cirrhosis. In a small percentage of affected individuals, more extensive multilobular cirrhosis develops. The gallbladder is frequently atrophic and filled with mucus. The cystic duct and the intrahepatic and extrahepatic ducts may be filled with mucus and sludge.

The vas deferens is occluded in almost all males with CF. Thus, virtually all males with CF are sterile. In females, increased viscosity of cervical mucus has been described. Pathology is minimal, however. Healthy females with CF successfully conceive and are capable of carrying pregnancies to term. (*From* Forstner and Durie [15]; with permission.)

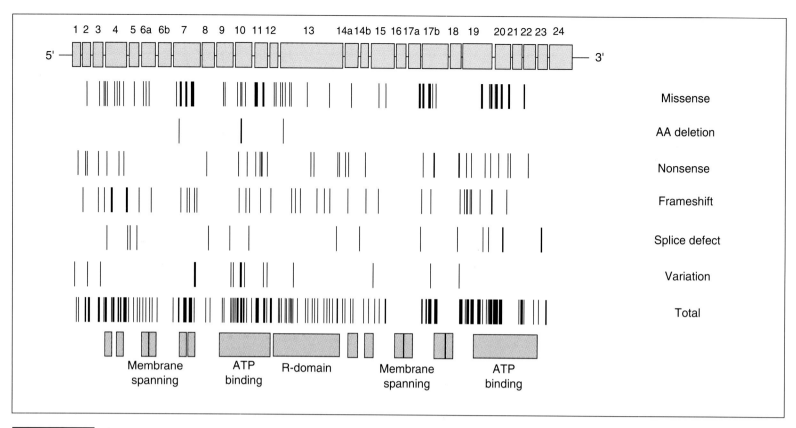

FIGURE 9-6.

Distribution of cystic fibrosis transmembrane conductance regulator (CFTR) gene mutations. The predominant mutation that causes cystic fibrosis (ΔF508) accounts for approximately 70% of mutant chromosomes screened [18]. Under the leadership of Dr. L.-C. Tsui, the Cystic Fibrosis Genetic Analysis Consortium was formed in 1989 to pool knowledge and information concerning CFTR gene mutations. To date the Consortium has identified more than 500 sequence alterations. Most of these mutations are almost certainly associated with the disease. The distribution and nature of the mutations in the CFTR gene are shown. The boxes at the top represent exons; the functional domains of the CFTR protein are shown at the bottom. Each vertical bar shows the location of a mutation reported to the CF Genetic Analysis Consortium (as of May 1992). A variation suggests a benign amino acid substitution. (*From* Tsui [19]; with permission.)

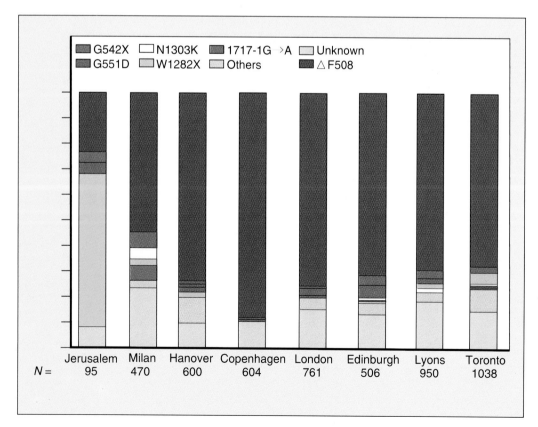

FIGURE 9-7.

The relative frequencies of the common cystic fibrosis transmembrane conductance regulator (CFTR) gene mutations in selected population centers are shown. A founder effect is apparent for some of the more common mutations. For example, ΔF508 accounts for almost 90% of CFTR mutations detected in the Danish population, suggesting that this mutation originated in Northeastern Europe. In contrast, ΔF508 accounts for only 22% of the cystic fibrosis chromosomes in the Ashkenazi Jewish population living in Israel. In that population, the nonsense mutation W1282X is common. It should be noted that a number of mutations remain unknown. (*Adapted from* Tsui [19]; with permission.)

TABLE 9-2. CLINICAL CHARACTERISTICS OF 293 PATIENTS ACCORDING TO GENOTYPE AND PANCREATIC-FUNCTION STATUS*

CHARACTERISTIC	ΔF508/ΔF508		ΔF508/OTHER		OTHER/OTHER	
	PI	PS	PI	PS	PI	PS
Patients, no	149	2	84	33	9	16
Patients with meconium ileus, %	22 (15)	0	10 (12)	0	4 (44)	0
Age at diagnosis, yr[†]	1.8±3.3	0.6±0.1	2.8±4.1[‡]	8.4±7.6	4.2±10.2[‡]	11±6
Sweat chloride level at diagnosis, mmol/L[†]	106±16	112±15	108±18[‡]	94±18	115±15[‡]	89±15
Current age, yr[†]	17±10	10±6	18±11[‡]	26±9	11±11[‡]	23±9
Current weight percentile[†]	39±30	32±2	42±31[‡]	64±29	31±31[‡]	73±19
Current height percentile	40±28	73±12	45±28	50±26	44±35	55±21
Current weight for height, %[†]	100±12	86±2	98±14[‡]	108±15	95±8[‡]	110±15

*PI denotes pancreatic insufficiency, and PS pancreatic sufficiency. Plus-minus values are means ±SD.
[†]P<0.001 by analysis of variance of five means (group in which n = 2 was not included in analysis).
[‡]Significantly different from the value for patients with pancreatic sufficiency within each genotype group (P<0.05, with Bonferroni's correction).

TABLE 9-2.

Clinical characteristics. Coincident with the accumulation of knowledge of cystic fibrosis transmembrane conductance regulator (CFTR) gene mutations, clinicians have gained considerable insight into genotype-phenotype relationships. Among the various clinical findings, the most striking association is with the presence or absence of pancreatic insufficiency. Of patients with cystic fibrosis, 293 were evaluated for the presence of the most common CFTR gene mutation (ΔF508); the results were compared with the clinical manifestations of the disease [20]. Of the patients, 52% were homozygous for the mutation, 40% were heterozygous, and 8% had other undefined mutations. The patients who are homozygous for the mutation had been diagnosed as having cystic fibrosis at an early age; in 99% of these patients pancreatic insufficiency was present. In contrast, only 72% of the heterozygous patients and 36% of the patients with other genotypes had pancreatic insufficiency. Patients with pancreatic insufficiency in all three genotype groups had similar clinical characteristics, reflected by an earlier diagnosis, similar sweat chloride values at diagnosis, similar severity of pulmonary disease, and similar percentile for weight. By comparison, the heterozygous-genotype and other genotype groups that did not have pancreatic insufficiency were older and had milder disease. They had lower sweat chloride values at diagnosis, normal nutritional status, and as a group, pulmonary function was better after adjustment for age. (*Adapted from* Kerem *et al.* [20]; with permission.)

PANCREATIC INSUFFICIENCY

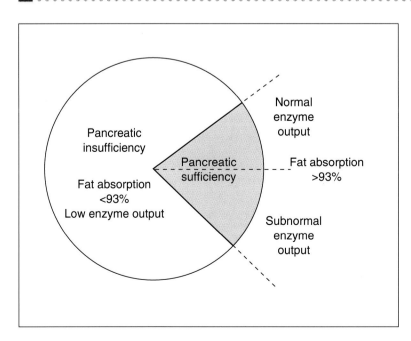

FIGURE 9-8.

The term *pancreatic insufficiency* describes patients who have evidence of maldigestion due to pancreatic failure. Those who absorb fat normally are often said to have normal pancreatic function, but when evaluated by quantitative measure of pancreatic function, they frequently have exocrine function that is below the normal level. It seems appropriate to use the term *pancreatic sufficiency* to define a patient who lacks steatorrhea and does not require pancreatic enzymes with meals. Overall prognosis and management of the patients with pancreatic sufficiency are somewhat different from that of patients with pancreatic insufficiency. Pancreatic sufficiency is an operational term and does not imply that the ability to secrete anions, fluid, and zymogens is normal. (*Adapted from* Forstner and Durie [15].)

TABLE 9-3. CLASSIFICATION OF CF GENE MUTATIONS AS SEVERE OR MILD WITH RESPECT TO PANCREATIC FUNCTION

Type of mutation	Severe (location)	Mild (location)
Missense (point mutation)	I148T (exon 4)	R117H (exon 4)
	G480C (exon 9)	R334W (exon 7)
	V520F (exon 10)	
	G551D (exon 11)	R347P (exon 7)
	R560T (exon 11)	A455E (exon 9)
	N1303K (exon 21)	P574H (exon 12)
Single amino acid deletion	ΔF508 (exon 10)	
	ΔI507 (exon 10)	
Stop codon (nonsense)	Q493X (exon 10)	
	G542X (exon 11)	
	R553X (exon 11)	
	W1282X (exon 20)	
Splice junction	621 + 1G → T (intron 4)	
	1717-1G → T (intron 10)	
Frameshift	556delA (exon 4)	
	3659delC (exon 19)	

TABLE 9-3.

Investigations of families with more than one affected member showed that the presence of pancreatic sufficiency or pancreatic insufficiency is highly concordant within families [21]. To evaluate the genetic basis of this observation, complete genotypes were determined in 394 patients in whom pancreatic status was well documented. The data showed that, with very few exceptions, each genotype was associated with pancreatic insufficiency only or with pancreatic sufficiency only. This finding is consistent with the hypothesis that the pancreatic function phenotype is determined by the genotype at the cystic fibrosis transmembrane conductance regulator (CFTR) gene locus. More specifically, the pancreatic sufficiency phenotype occurs in patients carrying one or two "mild" CFTR gene mutations, whereas the pancreatic insufficiency phenotype occurs in patients with two "severe" alleles. All the nonsense (stop codon), splice junction, and frameshift mutations were "severe" with respect to pancreatic function status. ΔF508 and ΔI507, which are single amino acid deletions, are also severe with respect to the pancreas. Interestingly, the study showed that missense mutations (amino acid substitutions) could be either severe or mild. (*Adapted from* Kristidis *et al.* [22]; with permission.)

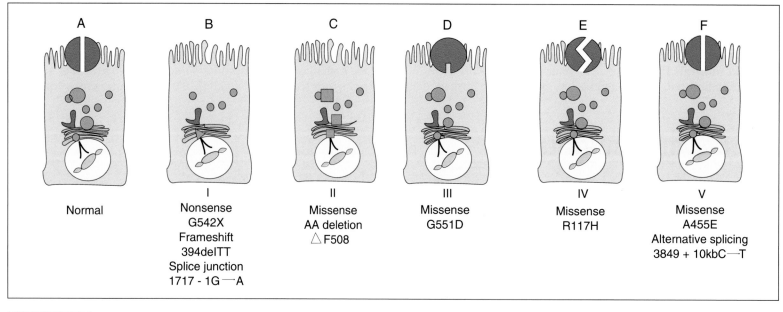

A Normal

B I Nonsense G542X Frameshift 394delTT Splice junction 1717 - 1G → A

C II Missense AA deletion △F508

D III Missense G551D

E IV Missense R117H

F V Missense A455E Alternative splicing 3849 + 10kbC—T

FIGURE 9-9.

Attempts have been made to define the different mutations into classes according to the functional properties of the gene product with respect to chloride regulation. A modified classification system, originally proposed by Tsui [19], is shown. **A,** Normal mutations. **B,** Class I represents gene mutations for which the intact cystic fibrosis transmembrane conductance regulator (CFTR) protein product is not formed. Most nonsense mutations fit into this category. **C,** Class II represents the forms of mutation CFTR that fail to traffic to the apical membrane under physiologic conditions. ΔF508 is the most striking example of this class of mutations. **D,** Class III mutant CFTR proteins include those that are inserted into the apical membrane but fail to respond to stimulation with cyclic adenosine monophosphate (cAMP). The relatively common missense mutation G551D is an example of a class III mutation. **E,** Class IV mutants produce protein that reach the apical membrane, generate cAMP-regulated apical membrane chloride current, but have altered channel properties, resulting in a reduction in the amount of current. Most mutations in this class are represented by the "mild" pancreatic sufficient CFTR gene mutations outlined in Table 9-3. **F,** Class V mutations are extremely rare. They result in reduced synthesis of normal functioning CFTR because of defective processing or aberrant splicing at alternative sites. Class IV and class V mutations have a strong association with the pancreatic sufficient phenotype. (*From* Wilchanski *et al.* [23]; with permission.)

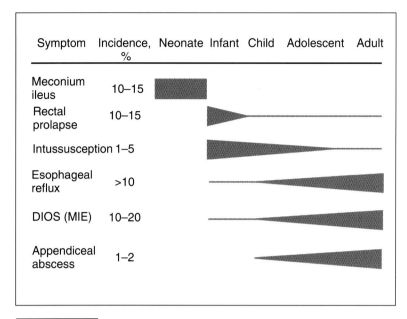

Symptom	Incidence, %	Neonate	Infant	Child	Adolescent	Adult
Meconium ileus	10–15					
Rectal prolapse	10–15					
Intussusception	1–5					
Esophageal reflux	>10					
DIOS (MIE)	10–20					
Appendiceal abscess	1–2					

FIGURE 9-10.

Gastrointestinal manifestations vary with age and disease progression. Approximately 10% to 15% of cystic fibrosis (CF) patients present at birth with signs and symptoms of intestinal obstruction. The cause is a plug of meconium in the terminal ileum that is acquired in utero. Half the cases are complicated by volvulus and atresia with or without attendant meconium peritonitis. Rectal prolapse occurs in almost 20% of patients, usually between 1 and 2.5 years of age [25]. In almost half these cases, episodes of prolapse precede diagnosis. Rectal prolapse has a tendency to resolve spontaneously.

Gastroesophageal reflux that may cause severe esophagitis and esophageal stricture increases in frequency with age, being more common in older children or adults with chronic pulmonary disease [26]. Distal intestinal obstruction syndrome (DIOS) or meconium ileus equivalent (MIE) occurs mainly in patients with pancreatic insufficiency [27]. It results from inspissated fecal masses that adhere tightly to the intestinal mucosa, particularly in the ileocecal area. An abdominal mass can be palpated in the abdomen. Complete bowel obstruction is rare; more often it causes partial bowel obstruction with intermittent abdominal pain that may result in loss of appetite and weight loss. Classical symptoms of acute appendicitis seem to be relatively rare in CF. More frequently, patients develop an appendicial abscess that is frequently misdiagnosed as DIOS.

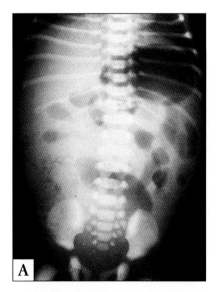

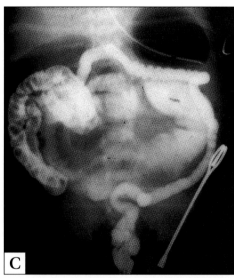

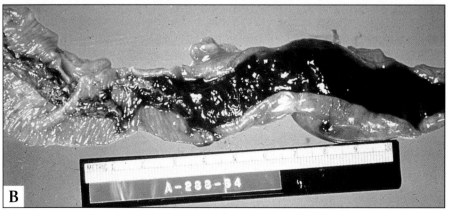

FIGURE 9-11.

Meconium ileus. **A,** A plain radiograph of the abdomen shows numerous gas-filled loops, displaced by meconium in the right lower quadrant. Small, multiple bubbles of gas are obvious within the meconium. No air is present in the rectum. **B,** Resected surgical specimen of the ileum from a patient with cystic fibrosis (CF) with meconium ileus. Rubbery, inspissated meconium is adherent to the intestinal mucosa (ileum is dissected open longitudinally). **C,** Water-soluble air contrast enema of a newborn with CF and complicated meconium ileas. A microcolon is demonstrated. Meconium plugs are shown in the ileum, which is opacified with contrast material. (**A,** *From* Forstner and Durie [15]; with permission.)

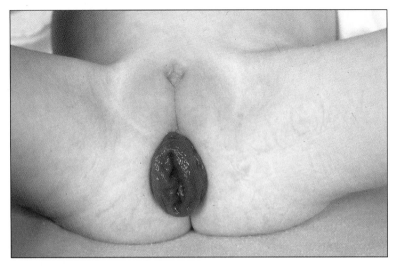

FIGURE 9-12.

Rectal prolapse, which usually occurs during passage of a large bowel motion, can be a frightening condition for parents of young children. It is hardly ever associated with major medical complications and is easily reduced manually. This condition usually resolves spontaneously by 3 to 4 years of age. Surgical intervention is not advocated, unless the condition is persistent.

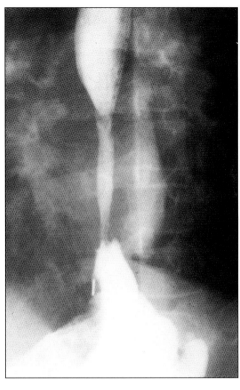

FIGURE 9-13.

A barium esophagogram in a 7-year-old girl with cystic fibrosis and advanced pulmonary disease. A severe distal esophageal stricture resulting from reflux esophagitis is demonstrated.

■ DISTAL INTESTINAL OBSTRUCTION SYNDROME

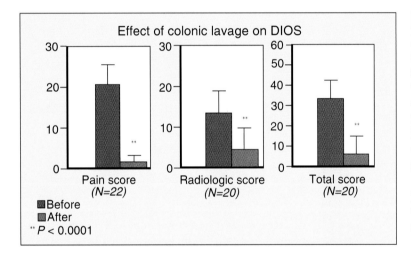

FIGURE 9-14.

Effect of colonic lavage on distal intestinal obstruction syndrome (DIOS). Episodes of DIOS are usually chronic and recurrent in the susceptible patient. Symptoms may be relieved by intestinal lavage with a balanced isotonic, polyethylene glycol-salt solution delivered orally or through a nasogastric tube. In patients with cystic fibrosis who sought medical attention for DIOS, treatment was initiated with the lavage solution. Although 14 patients chose to drink the solution, the 8 remaining patients elected to use a nasogastric tube. The solution was administered at the average rate of 1 liter per hour with an average volume of 5.6 liters. All but one patient reported impressive improvement when assessed by a semi-quantitative scoring system designed to assess the severity of pain and the degree of fecal impaction on plain abdominal radiograph [27]. (*Adapted from* Koletzko *et al.* [27]; with permission.)

HEPATOBILIARY DISEASE

TABLE 9-4. HEPATOBILIARY COMPLICATIONS OF CYSTIC FIBROSIS

HEPATIC COMPLICATIONS	REPORTED FREQUENCY, %
Neonatal cholestasis	Uncommon
Fatty liver	15–30
Focal biliary cirrhosis	11–70
Multilobular cirrhosis	2–5
Liver failure	Rare
BILIARY COMPLICATIONS	
Microgallbladder	5–20
Cholelithiasis	10
Intrahepatic biliary disease	Unknown
Extrahepatic biliary disease	Unknown
Common bile duct obstruction	Unknown

TABLE 9-4.

Liver disease, characterized by prolonged cholestatic jaundice, may be the presenting feature of cystic fibrosis (CF) in the neonate.

The onset may be delayed several weeks with manifestations suggestive of biliary atresia, but jaundice usually resolves spontaneously. Investigations usually focus on other causes of neonatal jaundice. Isolated hepatomegaly without cholestasis may also be seen in infancy and early childhood. This may result from steatosis when the liver is smooth, soft, and only moderately enlarged. The etiology and significance of hepatic steatosis in CF remain an enigma. Focal biliary cirrhosis is, by far, the most common hepatic complication; incidence as high as 70% is reported on postmortem examination. A small number of patients develop advanced multilobular cirrhosis with portal hypertension and hypersplenism. Hyperbilirubinemia is rare. Overt liver failure is an unusual complication in CF.

Abnormalities of the biliary tract are quite common. Patients frequently have nonfunctioning microgallbladders whereas others have distended gallbladders as if obstructed. Gallstones are common. Cholangiographic studies reveal abnormalities of both the intrahepatic and extrahepatic ducts in a large percentage of older patients. Common bile duct obstruction due to fibrosis of the head of the pancreas has been postulated as a major cause of CF-associated liver disease. Other studies have questioned the high prevalence of this abnormality. Intrahepatic and extrahepatic ductal filling defects appear to be present in a large percentage of patients. Some of these changes, which resemble sclerosing cholangitis, are probably due to intraluminal accumulation of sludge or protein and mucus. (*Adapted from* Forstner and Durie [15].)

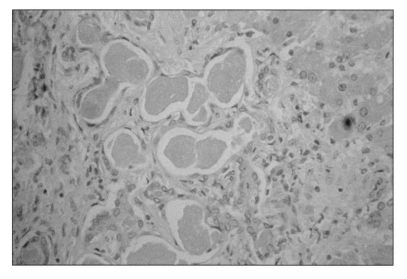

FIGURE 9-15.

A portal area from the liver biopsy of a patient with cystic fibrosis who also has focal biliary cirrhosis. Marked eosinophilic plugging of bile ductules is present. Bile ductules are increased in number and their cells are flattened. Periductal cell infiltration, bile duct proliferation, and increased fibrosis are common in scattered portal tracts. The patchy, focal nature of these lesions makes interpretation using needle liver biopsy to determine the severity of liver disease problematic. (*From* Forstner and Durie [15]; with permission.)

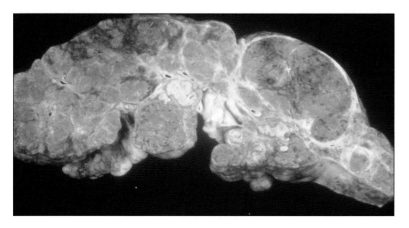

FIGURE 9-16.

Cut section of a postmortem liver from a patient with cystic fibrosis (CF) and multilobular cirrhosis. This patient had portal hypertension and hypersplenism. Gross cholestasis and nodular cirrhosis are present. Patients with advanced multilobular cirrhosis rarely die of hepatic failure. As life expectancy increases, however, clinical problems associated with CF liver disease, such as recurrent refractory variceal bleeding, hypersplenism, intractable ascites, and portosystemic encephalopathy will no doubt become more common. Some of these patients may be aided by hepatic transplantation.

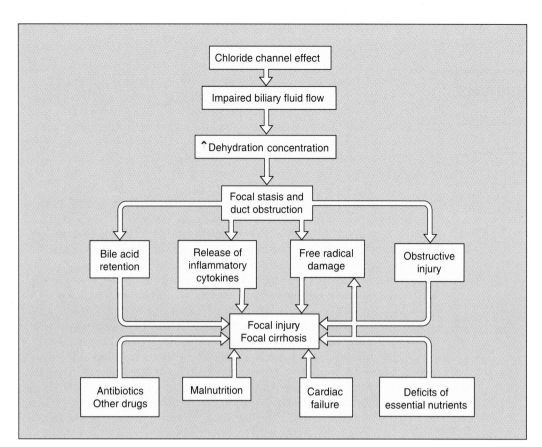

FIGURE 9-17.

Pathogenesis of hepatic injury. A variety of factors could contribute to hepatic injury and cystic fibrosis. The basic defect could result in reduced flow within small intrahepatic ducts. Mechanical obstruction caused by mucus plugs, intra- or extrahepatic lithiasis, distal stenosis of the common bile duct, or right cardiac failure could contribute to liver injury. Hepatotoxic factors include toxic bile acids together with various antibiotics and other pharmacotherapy. Free radical injury (with vitamin E deficiency), the presence of chronic malnutrition, or deficits of essential nutrients (fatty acids and taurine) might be expected to mediate hepatic injury as well.

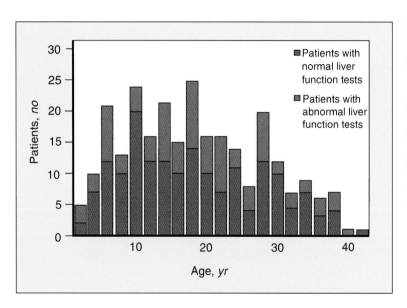

FIGURE 9-18.

No completely satisfactory methods exist for evaluating patients with cystic fibrosis (CF) for the presence or severity of liver disease [10]. Routine liver enzyme tests such as alkaline phosphatase and aspartate transaminase are mildly elevated in about 40% of CF patients. Liver enzyme test abnormalities are usually 150% to 200% higher than normal. The precise cause and significance of these abnormalities are unknown. Some patients with advanced multilobular cirrhosis can have normal results of routine liver tests. This figure shows the frequency of abnormal alkaline phosphatase with or without aspartate transaminase activities with age in patients who are homozygous for ΔF508.

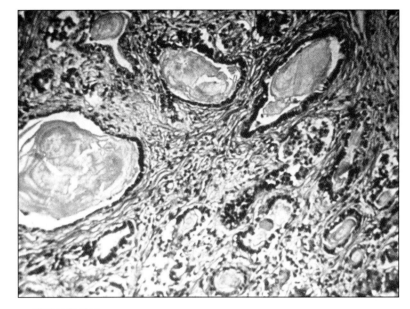

FIGURE 9-19.

Histologic section of a pancreas from a patient with cystic fibrosis. Pancreatic damage begins in utero with accumulation of protein-aceous secretory material within small pancreatic ducts [28]. The obstructive process causes dilatation of the duct lumina, which is followed by progressive degradation and atrophy of the acini. In patients with pancreatic insufficiency, advanced acinar destruction is present by the first few years of life and exocrine glands become replaced by fibrous tissue and fat. Initially, endocrine tissue is relatively preserved but as patients grow older islet cells are lost and the glands become completely replaced with fibrous tissue. Pancreatic calcification and cystic changes are occasionally seen in older patients.

TABLE 9-5. TESTS OF PANCREATIC FUNCTION

DIRECT	INDIRECT	BLOOD
Intubation tests	Stool microscopy	Pancreatic enzymes
Hormone stimulants	72-hr fecal fat	Pancreatic polypeptide
	Stool enzymes	
Natural stimulants	Bentiromide	
	Fluorescein dilaurate	
	Breath tests	

TABLE 9-5.

Diagnosis of pancreatic function status. Several indirect and direct tests of pancreatic function are available for defining pancreatic status. Simple methods such as microscopic examination of a stool smear for neutral fat droplets are helpful, but more quantitative methods, such as determining 72-hour fecal fat losses while the patient's fat intake is measured, can be used to define the presence or absence of pancreatic insufficiency. Deficient secretion of pancreatic enzymes in stool can be ascertained by analysis of stool chymotrypsin activity. Alternative, indirect tests of pancreatic function, such as bentiromide or fluorescein dilaurate, can be helpful for distinguishing pancreatic insufficient and pancreatic sufficient patients and for monitoring pancreatic function in those with pancreatic sufficiency. More complex direct intubation studies are of value for defining the residual pancreatic capacity of patients with pancreatic sufficiency.

FIGURE 9-20.

Sudan red stain for fecal fat in cystic fibrosis (CF). Stool smear of a patient with CF stained with sudan-red. Numerous stained fat droplets are seen.

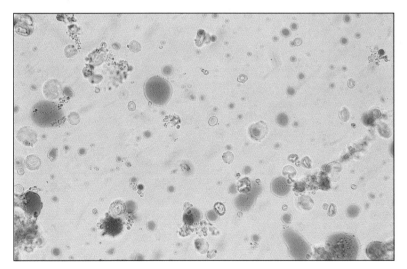

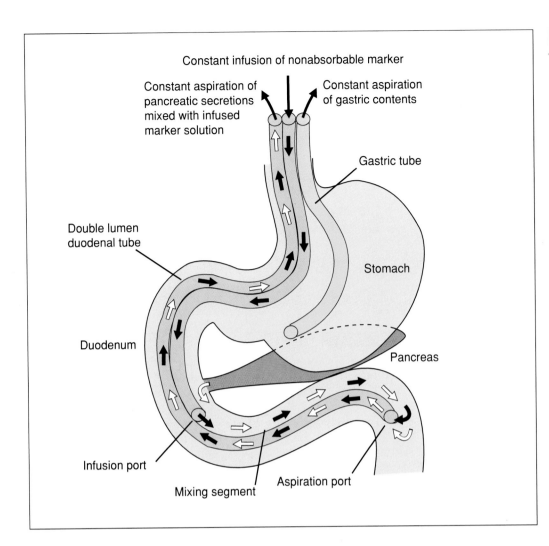

Constant infusion of nonabsorbable marker

Constant aspiration of pancreatic secretions mixed with infused marker solution

Constant aspiration of gastric contents

Gastric tube

Double lumen duodenal tube

Stomach

Duodenum

Pancreas

Infusion port

Aspiration port

Mixing segment

FIGURE 9-21.

The complex, direct method for assessing pancreatic function is represented diagrammatically. A double lumen tube is inserted into the duodenum. The tube is constructed so that one lumen opens proximally at the ampulla of Vater and the second lumen, which has several distal ports, is positioned distally at the ligament of Treitz. A nonabsorbable marker solution is infused into a proximal port at a constant rate. Pancreatic juice mixed with infused marker solution is aspirated distally by low-pressure suction. Following equilibration of marker solution with pancreatic juice, duodenal juice mixed with marker is collected while continuously and simultaneously infusing secretin and cholecystokinin at doses known to achieve maximal pancreatic stimulation. A separate nasogastric tube facilitates aspiration of gastric juice and minimizes contamination of duodenal contents with acid and pepsin. Use of a nonabsorbable marker permits correction for distal losses of fluid and enzyme by assuming that, after equilibration has been attained, the degree of distal loss of marker equals pancreatic enzyme and fluid loss. (*Adapted from* Couper *et al.* [29].)

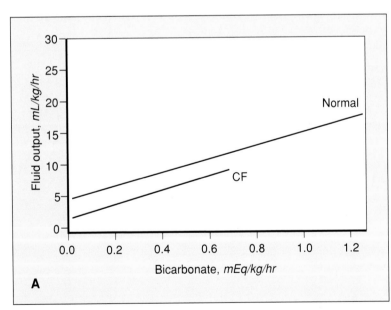

A

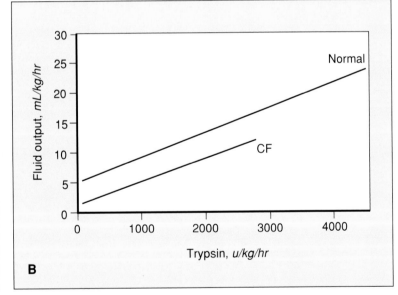

B

FIGURE 9-22.

A–B, The invasive, complex nature of the direct pancreatic function test tends to discourage its routine use. It is particularly helpful, however, for diagnosing cystic fibrosis (CF) or excluding the diagnosis in difficult cases. Deficits in anion levels (chloride and bicarbonate) and fluid secretion in CF compared with normal controls provide evidence of the underlying defect within epithelial cells of the pancreatic duct. (*Adapted from* Kopelman *et al.* [17].)

Range of pancreatic function

100% ← — — — — → 1% ← — — → 0%

Pancreatic sufficiency   Pancreatic insufficiency

FIGURE 9-23.

The direct pancreatic function test is helpful in delineating the pancreatic reserve in patients who are pancreatically sufficient. More than 98% of exocrine pancreatic capacity must be lost before signs and symptoms of steatorrhea develop.

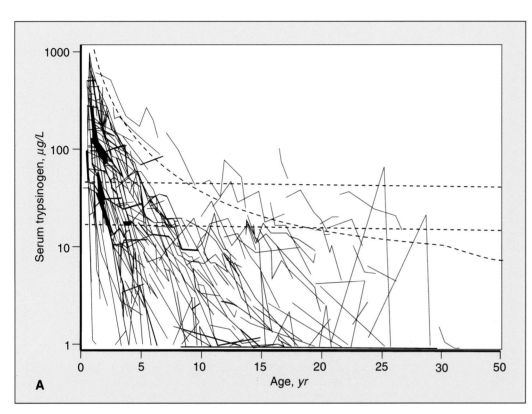

A

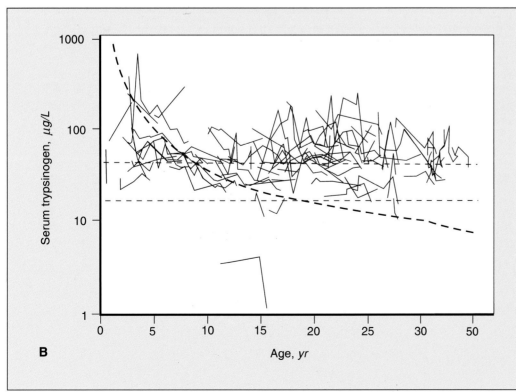

B

FIGURE 9-24.

Pancreatic enzymes, such as trypsinogen, can be detected in sera by immunologic techniques. This technique can be used to define pancreatic disease in cystic fibrosis (CF). Serum trypsinogen levels are greatly elevated in the blood of newborn infants with CF, presumably because of an obstruction of the small pancreatic ducts and regurgitation of pancreatic enzymes into the circulation. This test is used for screening neonates for CF. Longitudinal monitoring of serum trypsinogen can also be useful for predicting loss of pancreatic function. **A,** Serial measurements of serum trypsinogen in 233 patients with CF and pancreatic insufficiency. *Parallel dotted lines* indicate the normal range of values. The *curved dotted line* indicates the upper limits (95% confidence limits) for pancreatically insufficient measurements. As the pancreas atrophies, serum trypsinogen values drop, reaching subnormal values in patients by 7 to 8 years of age. **B,** Serial measurements of serum trypsinogen in 78 patients with CF and pancreatic sufficiency. The *parallel dotted lines* indicate the normal range of values. The *curved dotted line* indicates the upper limits (95% confidence limits) for the patients with pancreatic insufficiency. Most patients show widely fluctuating values within or above the normal range. One patient with unusually low results of a serum trypsinogen test died of gastrointestinal lymphoma.

TABLE 9-6. CLINICAL SIGNS OF MALNUTRITION IN CYSTIC FIBROSIS

In infancy and childhood	In late childhood and adolescence
Growth retardation	Growth retardation
Delayed bone age	Weight deficit
Weight deficit	Muscle wasting
Muscle wasting	Delayed puberty
Pot belly	Hepatomegaly
Rectal prolapse	Hypoalbuminemia
Hypoalbuminemia	Osteopenia
Edema	Ataxia
Anemia	Ophthalmoplegia
Bruising	
Bleeding	
Skin rash	
Hepatomegaly	
Developmental delay	

TABLE 9-6.

Clinical features of malnutrition. Signs and symptoms of malnutrition vary according to the patient's age, but most are related to a protein-calorie deficit or malabsorption of essential nutrients [15]. Most patients with cystic fibrosis (CF) and pancreatic insufficiency present in infancy with some manifestations of maldigestion and are often malnourished. The abdomen is distended and muscles appear wasted, particularly in the buttocks and thighs. Growth failure is an early sign. The appearance of edema, hypoalbuminemia, and anemia herald severe protein-calorie malnutrition; this generally occurs in infants under the age of 6 months. Growth retardation is a variable feature during childhood. In general, patients improve rapidly with adequate attention to caloric requirements, vitamin needs, and pancreatic enzyme supplementation. In most CF centers, nutritional support is now viewed as an integral part of the multidisciplinary care of patients with CF. Aggressive programs have been instituted to prevent malnutrition. It is now generally accepted that the primary objective of nutritional management is to achieve normal nutrition and growth for children of all ages.

TABLE 9-7. DISORDERS CAUSED BY DEFICITS OF ESSENTIAL NUTRIENTS

Fat-soluble vitamin deficiency	
A	Raised intracranial pressure
	Conjunctival xerosis
	Night blindness
D	Rickets
	Osteomalacia
E	Hemolytic anemia (infants)
	Neuropathy
	Ophthalmoplegia
	Ataxia
	Diminished vibration sense and proprioception
K	Coagulopathy
Water-soluble vitamin deficiency	B_{12} deficiency in PI patients not receiving or non-compliant to enzyme therapy
Salt depletion	Lethargy
	Weakness
	Dehydration
	Metabolic alkalosis
Essential fatty acid deficiency	Desquamation
	Thrombocytopenia
	Poor wound healing

TABLE 9-7.

Deficits of essential nutrients. Fat-soluble vitamin deficiencies caused by malabsorption are common in untreated pancreatically insufficient (PI) patients. These include night blindness, ataxia, and neuropathy. Deficiencies of water-soluble vitamins are rare. Vitamin deficiencies are preventable with appropriate therapy (pancreatic enzymes and supplemental fat-soluble vitamins). Salt depletion, because of excessive sweating, particularly in hotter climates, may cause symptoms of hyponatremia. Signs and symptoms of essential fatty acid deficiency may be present before diagnosis but are rare in nourished, appropriately treated, patients. Biochemical evidence of essential fatty acid deficiency may persist following therapy, however.

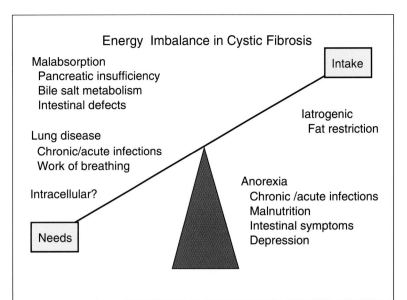

Energy Imbalance in Cystic Fibrosis

Malabsorption
  Pancreatic insufficiency
  Bile salt metabolism
  Intestinal defects

Lung disease
  Chronic/acute infections
  Work of breathing

Intracellular?

Needs

Intake

Iatrogenic
  Fat restriction

Anorexia
  Chronic /acute infections
  Malnutrition
  Intestinal symptoms
  Depression

FIGURE 9-25.

Pathogenesis of energy imbalance in cystic fibrosis (CF). Various complex-related and unrelated factors may give rise to energy imbalance in patients with CF [11]. The net effect on growth potential varies from patient to patient, according to differences in disease expression and with disease progression. Expressed in simple terms, an energy deficit results from an imbalance between energy needs and intake, which in turn is determined by three factors: energy losses, energy expenditure, and energy intake.

TABLE 9-8. ENERGY IMBALANCE CAUSED BY CYSTIC FIBROSIS

INCREASED NEEDS	REDUCED INTAKE
Increased intestinal losses	Reduced intake
Pancreatic insufficiency	Iatrogenic fat
Bile salt metabolism	Anorexia
Hepatobiliary disease	Feeding disorders
Regurgitation from	Depression
gastroesophageal reflux	Esophagitis
Increased urinary losses	
Diabetes mellitus	
Increased energy expenditure	
Pulmonary disease	
Primary defect?	

TABLE 9-8.

Causes of energy imbalance in cystic fibrosis (CF). Fecal nutrient losses from maldigestion and malabsorption are known to contribute to energy imbalance. Despite improvements in the enzymatic potency and intestinal delivery of ingested pancreatic enzyme supplements, many patients continue to have severe maldigestion even when treated with adequate amounts of enzymes. Calorie restriction, especially with reduced dietary fat to relieve symptoms, may cause energy imbalance and adversely affect growth. It is suggested that energy intakes in cystic fibrosis exceed normal requirements, but in reality energy needs are extremely variable. Some patients with CF do have a higher energy expenditure than normal. Some studies have hinted at the possibility that the CF gene might have a direct effect on basal metabolism. Conversely, chest infections with or without inflammatory mediators or the energy expended in breathing may also raise energy expenditure. Patients with CF are prone to psychologic and gastrointestinal complications that might limit oral intake.

TABLE 9-9. GENETIC DEFECTS AND RESTING ENERGY EXPENDITURE IN CYSTIC FIBROSIS

	ΔF508/ ΔF508	ΔF508/ OTHER	OTHER/ OTHER
n	31	29	18
REE, % predicted	121	109	104
FEV$_1$	56	63	97

TABLE 9-9.

To evaluate the possibility that the genetic defect in cystic fibrosis (CF) has a direct effect on basal metabolism, O'Rawe and colleagues [30] demonstrated evidence of increased resting energy expenditure (REE) in patients homozygous for the most common CF trans-membrane conductance regulator gene mutation (ΔF508). In contrast, energy expenditure was only moderately increased in those with ΔF508/other and other/other genotypes. These investigators did not control for lung function or nutritional status, both of which could affect energy expenditure. Lung disease or lung infection increases REE; undernutrition may result in a decreased REE. (*Adapted from* O'Rawe *et al.* [30].) FEV$_1$—forced expiratory volume in 1 second.

TABLE 9-10. ENERGY EXPENDITURE AND LUNG DISEASE IN CYSTIC FIBROSIS

	ΔF508/ ΔF508 PI	ΔF508/ OTHER PI	F508/ OTHER PS
n	14	9	9
WFH, %	103	106	116
Body Fat, %	16	14	16
FEV$_1$	94	98	90
REE, % predicted	104	105	101

TABLE 9-10.

In a separate study the two confounding variables (malnutrition and lung disease) were accounted for by study males with normal nutritional status and good lung function—forced expiratory volume in 1 second (FEV$_1$>75% predicted). Little, if any, increase in resting energy expenditure (REE) was seen in normally nourished males with cystic fibrosis (CF) with good lung function [31]. Furthermore, we were unable to demonstrate any difference in REE in patient groups with different genotypes. Thus, if there is a genetic basis for increased REE in patients with CF, its effects must be minimal. PI—pancreatic insufficiency; PS—pancreatic sufficiency; WFH—weight as a percentage of ideal weight for height. (*Adapted from* Fried *et al.* [31].)

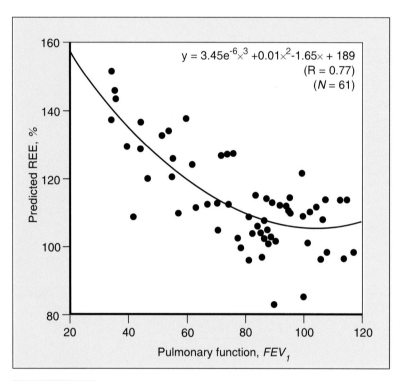

FIGURE 9-26.

Resting energy expenditure (REE) (as a percentage of predicted) versus pulmonary function in normally nourished males with cystic fibrosis. Lung function appears to be a major determinant of increased REE. As forced expiratory volume in 1 second (FEV$_1$) falls below 75% of predicted levels, REE rises in a curvilinear (quadratic) fashion, reaching values as high as 150% above predicted levels. At least two factors appear to affect REE. The first is a normal response to negative energy balance with a reduction in energy expenditure. The second, an increase in energy expenditure, appears to be related to the severity of lung function. The precise cause of increased resting energy expenditure remains to be elucidated. (*Adapted from* Fried *et al.* [31]; with permission.)

The equation shown in Figure 9-26:
$$y = 3.45e^{-6}x^3 + 0.01x^2 - 1.65x + 189$$
$$(R = 0.77)$$
$$(N = 61)$$

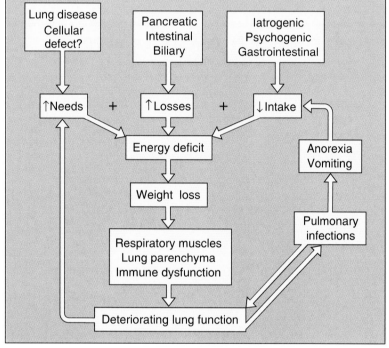

FIGURE 9-27.

Pathogenesis of an energy deficit. A proposed model to explain the cause of the energy deficit in patients with cystic fibrosis, which defines the web of independent and interdependent variables that may give rise to chronic malnutrition and growth failure. Most patients are able to maintain normal growth velocity and nutritional status by adherence to a good dietary routine, particularly when lung function is relatively unimpaired. Decline in pulmonary function and the development of malnutrition are closely interrelated, however. As lung function worsens, most commonly in adolescents and young adults, several factors may contribute to an energy deficit. More frequent and severe infections, coupled with the systemic effects of inflammatory mediators, may induce anorexia. Clinical depression, as a reaction to a chronic illness, may cause reduced intake. Weight loss causes loss of fat tissue and then muscle wasting. Respiratory muscle wasting could adversely affect respiratory motion, prevent effective coughing, and contribute to increasing lung disease. Malnutrition may impair immune function and lung elasticity. A vicious cycle is established wherein lowering lung function contributes to the nutritional deficit, which inevitably leads to endstage pulmonary failure and death. (*From* Durie and Pencharz [32]; with permission.)

REFERENCES

1. di Sant'Agnese P, Darling R, Perera G, Shea E: Abnormal electrolyte composition of sweat in cystic fibrosis of the pancreas. *Pediatrics* 1953, 12:549–563.

2. Fanconi G, Uehlinger E, Knauer C: Das Coelioksyndrom bei angeborener zystisher Pankreas Fibromatose and Bronchicktasis. *Wein Med Wochnenschr* 1936, 86:753–756.

3. Anderson D: Cystic fibrosis of the pancreas and its relation to celiac disease. *Am J Dis Child* 1938, 56:344–399.

4. Gibbs GE, Bostick WL, Smith PM: Incomplete pancreatic deficiency in cystic fibrosis of the pancreas. *J Pediatr* 1950, 37:320–325.

5. Quinton PM: Chloride impermeability in cystic fibrosis. *Nature* 1983, 301:421–422.

6. Knowles MR, Gatzy JT, Boucher RC: Relative ion permeability of normal and cystic fibrosis nasal epithelium. *J Clin Invest* 1983, 71:1410–1417.

7. Sato K, Sato F: Defective beta adrenergic response of cystic fibrosis sweat glands in vivo and in vitro. *J Clin Invest* 1984, 73:1763–1771.

8. Riordan JR, Rommens JM, Kerem BS, *et al.*: Identification of the cystic fibrosis gene: Cloning and characterization of complementary DNA. *Science* 1989, 245:1066–1073.

9. Bear CE, Li C, Kartner N, *et al.*: Purification and functional reconstitution of the cystic fibrosis transmembrane conductance regulator (CFTR). *Cell* 1992, 68:809–818.

10. Durie PR: Cystic fibrosis: Gastrointestinal and hepatic complications and their management. *Semin Pediatr Gastroenterol Nutr* 1993, 4:3.

11. Pencharz PB, Durie PR: Nutritional management of cystic fibrosis. *Annu Rev Nutr* 1993, 13:111–136.

12. Corey ML: Longitudinal studies in cystic fibrosis. In *Perspectives in Cystic Fibrosis*. Edited by Sturgess J. Proceedings of the Eighth International Congress in Cystic Fibrosis. Mississauga, Ontario, Canada: Imperial Press; 1980:246.

13. Gaskin K, Gurwitz D, Durie PR, *et al.*: Improved respiratory prognosis in patients with cystic fibrosis with normal fat absorption. *J Pediatr* 1982, 100:857–862.

14. Tsui L-C: The cystic fibrosis transmembrane conductance regulator gene. *Am J Respir Crit Care Med* 1995, 151:547–553.

15. Forstner G, Durie PR: Cystic fibrosis. In *Pediatric Gastrointestinal Disease. Pathophysiology, Diagnosis, Management*. Edited by Walker WA, Durie PR, Hamilton JR,et al. Philadelphia: BC Decker; 1991: 1179–1197.

16. Kopelman H, Durie PR, Gaskin K, *et al.*: Pancreatic fluid secretion and protein hyperconcentration in cystic fibrosis. *N Engl J Med* 1985, 312:329–334.

17. Kopelman H, Corey M, Gaskin K, *et al*: Impaired chloride secretion as well as bicarbonate secretion underlies the fluid secretory defect in the cystic fibrosis pancreas. *Gastroenterol* 1988, 95:349–355.

18. Kerem BS, Rommens JM, Buchanan JA, *et al.*: Identification of the cystic fibrosis gene: Genetic analysis. *Science* 1989, 245:1073–1080.

19. Tsui L-C: The spectrum of cystic fibrosis mutations. *Trends Genet* 1992, 8:392–398.

20. Kerem E, Corey M, Kerem B-S, *et al.*: The relation between genotype and phenotype in cystic fibrosis—analysis of the most common mutation (ΔF508). *N Engl J Med* 1990, 323:1517–1522.

21. Corey M, Durie PR, Moore D, *et al.*: Familial concordance of pancreatic function in cystic fibrosis. *J Pediatr* 1989, 115:274–277.

22. Kristidis P, Bozon D, Corey M, *et al.*: Genetic determination of exocrine pancreatic function in cystic fibrosis. *Am J Hum Genet* 1992, 50:1178–1184.

23. Wilchanski M, Zielenski J, Markiewicz D, *et al.*: Correlation of sweat chloride concentration classes of the cystic fibrosis transmembrane conductance regulator gene mutations. *J Pediatr* 1995, 127:705–710.

24. Kerem E, Corey M, Kerem B, *et al.*: Clinical and genetic comparisons of patients with cystic fibrosis, with or without meconium ileus. *J Pediatr* 1989, 114:767–773.

25. Stern R, Izant RJ, Boat TF, *et al.*: Treatment and prognosis of rectal prolapse in cystic fibrosis. *Gastroenterology* 1986, 82:707–710.

26. Scott RB, O'Laughlin EV, Gall DG: Gastroesophageal reflux in patients with cystic fibrosis. *J Pediatr* 1985, 106:223–227.

27. Koletzko S, Stringer DA, Cleghorn GJ, Durie PR: Lavage treatment of distal intestinal obstruction syndrome in children with cystic fibrosis. *Pediatrics* 1989, 83:727–733.

28. Oppenheimer E, Esterly J: Cystic fibrosis of the pancreas. *Arch Pathol Lab Med* 1973, 96:149–154.

29. Couper R, Durie P: Pancreatic function tests. In *Pediatric Gastrointestinal Disease. Pathophysiology, Diagnosis, Management*. Edited by Walter WA, Durie PR, Hamilton JR, *et al*. Philadelphia: BC Decker; 1991; 1341–1353.

30. O'Rawe A, McIntosh I, Dodge J, *et al*: Increased energy expenditure in cystic fibrosis is associated with specific mutations. *Clin Sci* 1992, 82:71–76.

31. Fried MD, Durie PR, Tsui L-C, *et al.*: The cystic fibrosis gene and resting energy expenditure. *J Pediatr* 1991, 119:913–916.

32. Durie PR, Pencharz PB: A rational approach to the nutritional care of patients with cystic fibrosis. *J R Soc Med* 1989, 82(Suppl 16):11–20.

Chapter 10

Hereditary Pancreatitis

DAVID C. WHITCOMB

Discovery of the mechanism that causes hereditary pancreatitis has been one of the most important recent findings in pancreatic diseases because it provides fundamental insights into the cause of both acute and chronic pancreatitis. Hereditary pancreatitis is a rare, chronic, idiopathic inflammatory disorder affecting multiple family members over two or more generations [1]. Inheritance occurs as an autosomal dominant trait with variable expression. Nearly 100 kindreds have been reported worldwide since the genetic basis of this disorder was recognized by Comfort and Steinberg in 1952 [2]. Most of the families are white, but Asian and East Indian families have also been reported. The classic description includes recurrent episodes of pancreatitis since childhood, equal distribution by gender, a family history of pancreatitis, a high frequency of large, calcified stones in the pancreatic duct, and exclusion of other causes of pancreatitis.

Using genetic linkage analysis and positional cloning, a mutation causing hereditary pancreatitis was discovered in the cationic trypsinogen gene [3,4]. Discovery that a mutant form of trypsin resistant to intrapancreatic inactivation, which leads to typical acute and chronic pancreatitis, and predisposes to pancreatic cancer, provides key insights to all major forms of pancreatitis and other pancreatic diseases. This chapter covers clinical and scientific issues associated with discovery and implication of the hereditary pancreatitis gene.

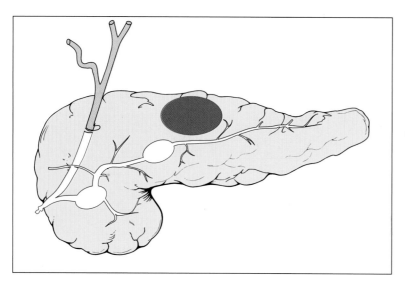

FIGURE 10-1.

Inflammatory diseases of the pancreas result in significant morbidity and mortality in patients throughout the world. In the past, various systems attempted to categorize pancreatitis according to dominant clinical, etiologic, or pathologic features. Today, however, most authorities simply divide these inflammatory conditions into acute (red area) or chronic (white area) pancreatitis. Through the study of hereditary pancreatitis, the link between these conditions is becoming clearer.

ACUTE AND CHRONIC PANCREATITIS

TABLE 10-1. PANCREATITIS: DEFINITION

Acute pancreatitis

Abdominal pain

Usually associated with elevated levels of pancreatic enzymes in blood or urine resulting from an inflammatory pancreatic disease

Chronic pancreatitis

Irreversible morphologic change, sclerosis

Pain

Permanent impairment of organ's function

TABLE 10-1.

Acute pancreatitis can be defined clinically as a condition typically presenting with abdominal pain, usually associated with elevated pancreatic enzymes in blood or urine owing to inflammation of the pancreas. *Chronic pancreatitis* can be defined as a continuous inflammatory disease of the pancreas characterized by irreversible morphologic change and typically causing pain with or without permanent impairment of function. Clinically, about 80% of patients present with recurrent or persistent abdominal pain. In more advanced stages of chronic pancreatitis, patients develop maldigestion or loss of endocrine function, leading to diabetes mellitus. Morphologically, the pancreas of patients with chronic pancreatitis show areas of fibrosis with loss of parenchyma in focal, segmental, or diffuse patterns; this loss is usually associated with ductal changes.

CLINICAL FINDINGS

TABLE 10-2. HEREDITARY PANCREATITIS: DEFINITION

Genetic predisposition

Autosomal dominant disorder

80% penetrance

Variable expressivity

Severe clinical features

Recurrent attacks of acute pancreatitis

Progression to chronic pancreatitis

High risk of pancreatic cancer

TABLE 10-2.

Hereditary pancreatitis is an unusual form of pancreatitis because it runs in families. This disorder is autosomal dominant in inheritance, with 80% penetrance worldwide.

Many patients affected by hereditary pancreatitis suffer a severe clinical course. Major features include recurrent attacks of acute pancreatitis, complications of chronic pancreatitis, and an increased risk of pancreatic cancer. Thus, the clinical features of hereditary pancreatitis encompass both acute and chronic pancreatitis.

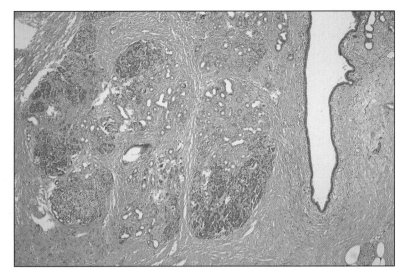

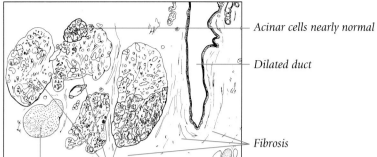

Acinar cells nearly normal

Dilated duct

Fibrosis

Islet of Langerhans   Loss of acinar cells from acinus

FIGURE 10-2.

Low-power histologic section from the pancreas of a patient with hereditary pancreatitis who underwent a Whipple operation. An enlarged pancreatic duct is indicated. Note the extensive fibrosis present with attendant loss of normal acinar cells. In addition, islets of Langerhans can be lost in the later stages of the disease process.

These changes are nonspecific and may be encountered in chronic pancreatitis resulting from other causes. Thus, the pathologic features of chronic hereditary pancreatitis are indistinguishable from chronic pancreatitis resulting from other etiologies indicated by histologic examination [5]. (Hematoxylin and eosin, original magnification × 40.)

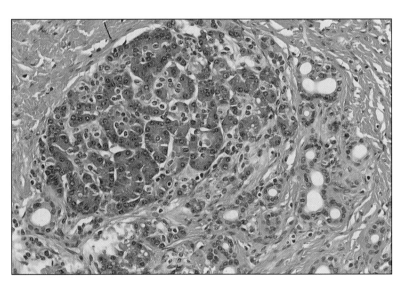

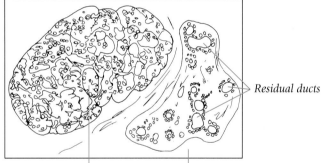

Residual ducts

Normal acinar cells   Loss of acinar cells

FIGURE 10-3.

Higher-power view of the pancreatic section shown in Figure 10-2. Note that a few normal-appearing acinar cells remain within the acinus on the left. Extensive fibrosis is present in the acinus on the right. Only residual pancreatic ducts remain present. (Hematoxylin and eosin, original magnification × 200.)

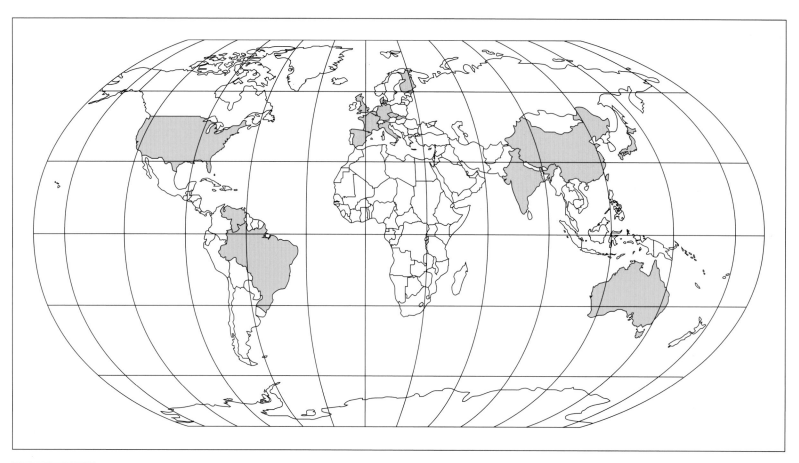

FIGURE 10-4.

Hereditary pancreatitis has been recognized worldwide. To date, most families have been of northern European descent; however, new families continue to emerge with better recognition of this disease. Comparison of the clinical features of these families has suggested that several milder forms may also exist, and the other mutations may also cause similar disease. In general, hereditary pancreatitis probably accounts for 1% to 2 % of all cases of acute and chronic pancreatitis.

TABLE 10-3. HEREDITARY PANCREATITIS: PROPOSED CAUSES

Hypertension in sphincter of Oddi

Altered pancreatic stone protein

Abnormal metabolism of lysine and cysteine

Structural malformation in ductal system

Deficiency of antioxidants (*eg*, glutathione, superoxide dismutase)

Human lymphocyte antigens (HLA) or immunologic disorder

TABLE 10-3.

Since the recognition of hereditary pancreatitis by Comfort and Steinberg in 1952, varied etiologies have been proposed. This table lists some of the most frequently cited theories, all of which have had some support; however, careful evaluation has excluded these from further consideration.

TABLE 10-4. ETIOLOGY OF HEREDITARY PANCREATITIS: IDENTIFICATION BY TRADITIONAL METHODS

No morphologic markers

No biochemical markers

Etiology unknown

TABLE 10-4.

Identification of the etiology of hereditary pancreatitis by traditional methods has been frustrating because in hereditary pancreatitis, no morphologic markers or biochemical markers are present. Therefore, the etiology of hereditary pancreatitis remained a mystery until 1996.

TABLE 10-5. HEREDITARY PANCREATITIS: GENETIC LINKAGE STUDY

Goal: Identification of *molecular* etiology
Method: Link disease to the disease gene
Requirement: Family with inherited phenotypic features
Not required: Morphologic markers, biochemical markers, mechanistic disease models

TABLE 10-5.

During the mid-1990s, several independent groups began using the evolving technology of molecular genetics to identify the cause of hereditary pancreatitis through genetic linkage studies. The goal of the genetics studies is to identify the molecular etiology of the disease. The method involves carefully identifying an inherited disease, then linking the disease to the disease's gene. The bases required for this type of study are a family within an inherited disease with well-defined phenotypic features. Neither morphologic or biochemical markers are required, nor is a mechanistic disease model.

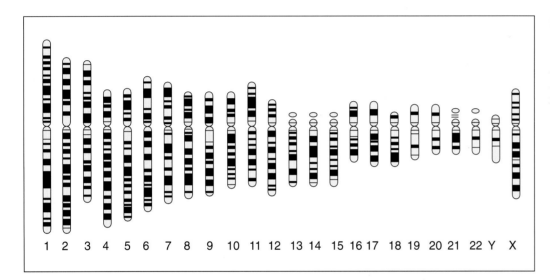

1 2 3 4 5 6 7 8 9 10 11 12 13 14 15 16 17 18 19 20 21 22 Y X

FIGURE 10-5.

Genetic linkage studies are powerful research tools because the primary molecular cause of the disease is identified. The problem is identifying the inherited mutation within the 3 billion DNA base pairs organized within the 23 pairs of human chromosomes.

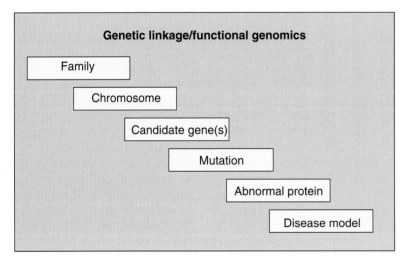

Genetic linkage/functional genomics

Family
Chromosome
Candidate gene(s)
Mutation
Abnormal protein
Disease model

FIGURE 10-6.

The process of identifying the cause of a disease by identifying abnormal genes is called *functional genomics*. In the study of hereditary pancreatitis, for example, this process went through six major steps. The first step is to identify and characterize a family. Once this was done, careful examination of markers on all 23 human chromosomes is made and compared with the inheritance of disease in the family. This identifies a single region of a chromosome that contains the affective gene. Once a region of a chromosome has been identified, candidate genes are examined. All genes that are expressed within this region are considered candidates. The candidate genes are analyzed for specific mutations. After the consistent mutation has been identified in all individuals affected with the disease, then the protein affected by the mutated gene codes can be identified. Then, after the abnormal protein has been identified, it is possible that the molecular model of the disease can be constructed.

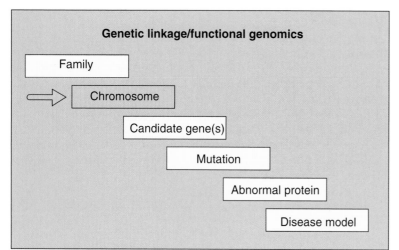

FIGURE 10-7.

One of the most important steps in the functional genomics process is to identify a region of a chromosome that contains the disease gene. This important step is reviewed here because it is central to identification of the gene causing hereditary pancreatitis.

GENETIC STUDIES

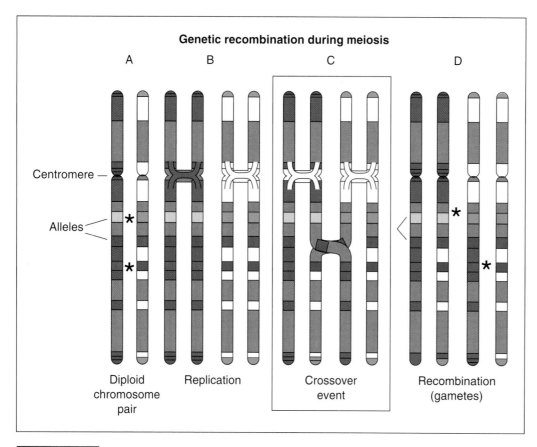

homologue; therefore, the organism has two copies of each gene. Identical sets of these chromosomes are present in all somatic cells. **B,** During replication, exact copies of each chromosome are made. In mitosis, the homologous pair of duplicate chromosomes remains independent, and one copy of each chromosome goes to the daughter cells during cell division to produce chromosomes identical to the original cell. **C,** During meiosis (leading to the sperm or the egg), the homologous pair of duplicated chromosomes lines up together. During this time, analogous portions of the chromosome's arms may crossover to the homologue's chromosome. The cell then divides twice without replication to form four gametes containing a single chromosome. **D,** As a result, the gamete shown on the right may have portions of the paternal chromosome and the maternal chromosome linked. Note the yellow and red markers on the brown chromosome in **part A.** Normally they would be transmitted together. Because a crossover event (**part C**) occurred between them, however, they are inherited separately in two of the gametes (**part D**), as shown by the stars. This crossover event is very important because it requires that each portion of each chromosome be identified and traced through the family tree, but it also allows precise localization of the disease gene, as is illustrated in the following figures.

FIGURE 10-8.

Major steps of meiosis leading to gametes (sperm and eggs), including genetic recombination [6]. It is this recombination that permits genetic mapping. **A,** On the left is a diploid set of chromosomes, one representing the maternal and the other representing the paternal

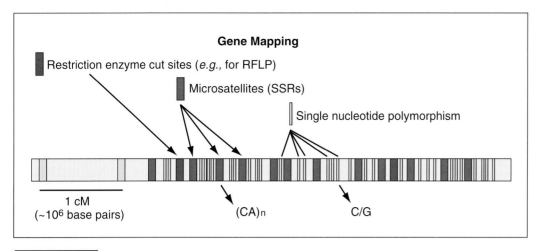

FIGURE 10-9.

One of the goals of the Human Genome Project was to develop a human genetic map with markers spaced every 2 to 5 centimorgan [6]. On genetic maps, the unit of distance is the centimorgan, representing a 1% chance of recombination within this region during a single meiosis. In other words, a 99% chance exists that this segment will stay together. On average, a centimorgan is about 1 million base pairs. Many markers have been identified, including restriction sites, microsatellites or simple sequence repeats (SSRs), and single nucleotide polymorphisms. The most useful markers for genetic mapping determined to date are microsatellites because they are of high density and many of them are hypervariable loci. High-density maps of single nucleotide polymorphisms are being developed and may become more useful in the future.

Microsatellites are made up of various identical sequences jointed in tandem. The most common is a CA repeat, in which CA refers to cytosine and adenosine, two of the four nucleotides that make up DNA. The CA repeats occur in 100,000 blocks in the human genome. They appeared to be present every 50,000 to 100,000 bases. In a particular microsatellite sequence, the CA will be repeated from 4 to 40 times. The longer sequences tend to be polymorphic in length, and therefore can be tracked through a family tree based on size, as illustrated in subsequent figures. RFLP—restriction fragment-length polymorphism.

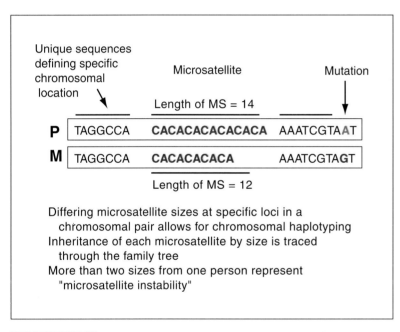

FIGURE 10-10.

Microsatellite. Note that there are two sections of DNA: one from the paternal side (labeled P) and the other from the maternal side (labeled M). The CA (cytosine-adenosine) repeats are shown in red and green. Notice also that whereas the length of the paternal microsatellite is 14 base pairs (bp), the microsatellite in the same location from the maternal side is only 12 bp, as is common in a hypervariable locus. This specific microsatellite can be distinguished from all other microsatellites by its flanking sequences. Notice that the flanking sequence on the left, TAGGCCA, is identical in the paternal and maternal chromosomes, and that this identifies this particular microsatellite at a specific location on a chromosome. The unique sequences that defined the chromosomal location can be used to develop polymerase chain reaction (PCR) primers so that the entire microsatellite can be amplified and the lengths of the microsatellite accurately measured on a sizing gel. Therefore, differing microsatellite sizes at specific location in a chromosomal pair allows for chromosomal haplotyping. In other words, the inheritance of each microsatellite can be traced through the entire family tree according to size. The reason this is improtant is that by sequentially looking at a large number of microsatellites that span the 23 chromosomal pairs, a microsatellite will be identified that is very close to the mutation that causes the inherited disease of interest. In this figure there is a guanine-to-adenine mutation in the parental chromosome very close to the microsatellite. Therefore, the mutation will be inherited through the family tree in a pattern similar to the microsatellite of 14 bp.

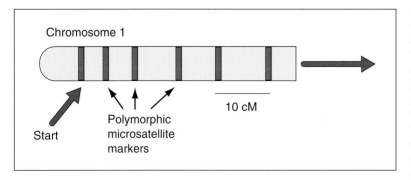

FIGURE 10-11.

A search for the mutant disease-causing gene can be conducted using variable microsatellite markers. A chromosome (eg, chromosome 1) is chosen to begin a genome-wide search. Markers that are polymorphic in size are then chosen every 5 to 10 centimorgans (cM). The marker is sized for each individual in the family and the inheritance pattern of the first marker is compared with the inheritance of the disease. If the inheritance pattern of the microsatellite and the disease are different, then the next marker is examined until a marker is found that is inherited in a matter identical to the disease. The marker and the disease are therefore linked. Because approximately 3 billion base pairs exist within the human genome, the genome can be completely screened with 300 to 400 markers spaced at 10-cM intervals.

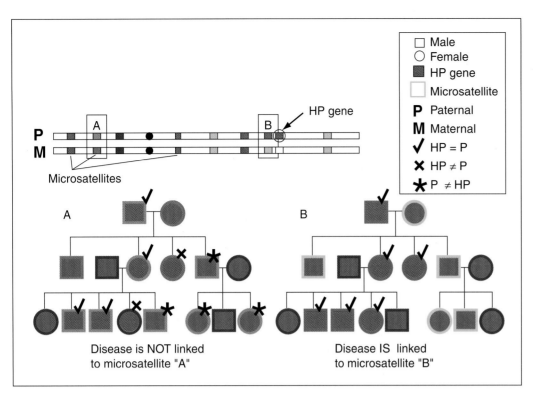

FIGURE 10-12.

The inheritance of microsatellite markers and a disease gene. Notice two chromosomes on the top left, the paternal (P) and maternal (M) chromosomes. Microsatellite A is considered first; microsatellite B second. Along the bottom of this figure is an illustration of a portion of the pedigree. The disease gene, in this case hereditary pancreatitis, is shown in bright green. In the first generation the grandfather was affected; in the second generation there were two affected daughters; in the third generation there were two affected sons and an affected daughter. The identical pedigree showing inheritance of the disease and the shown microsatellite marker at B.

Microsatellite marker A from the paternal chromosome is shown in orange. Notice that the affected grandfather's first child (far left) inherited microsatellite marker from the mother and did not have the disease. Likewise, the second child, a daughter, inherited the orange microsatellite marker A and also inherited hereditary pancreatitis; therefore, they match (shown with a check). The third child had hereditary pancreatitis but inherited the purple marker A from the mother, so the disease and the marker are *not* linked. The final child inherited the orange marker A from the father, but did not develop the disease; therefore it was not linked. Note that the oldest affected daughter was married and had five children. Again, inheritance of the disease is not linked to the inheritance of microsatellite marker A.

Consider microsatellite marker B on the chromosome at the top. Notice how closely the gene for hereditary pancreatitis appears in relation to marker B. In this case, the disease is linked to microsatellite marker B. The relationship of the mother to her five children in this pedigree should be noted, as well as an unaffected daughter, the next three affected children, and finally, an unaffected son. This is further investigated in Figure 10-13.

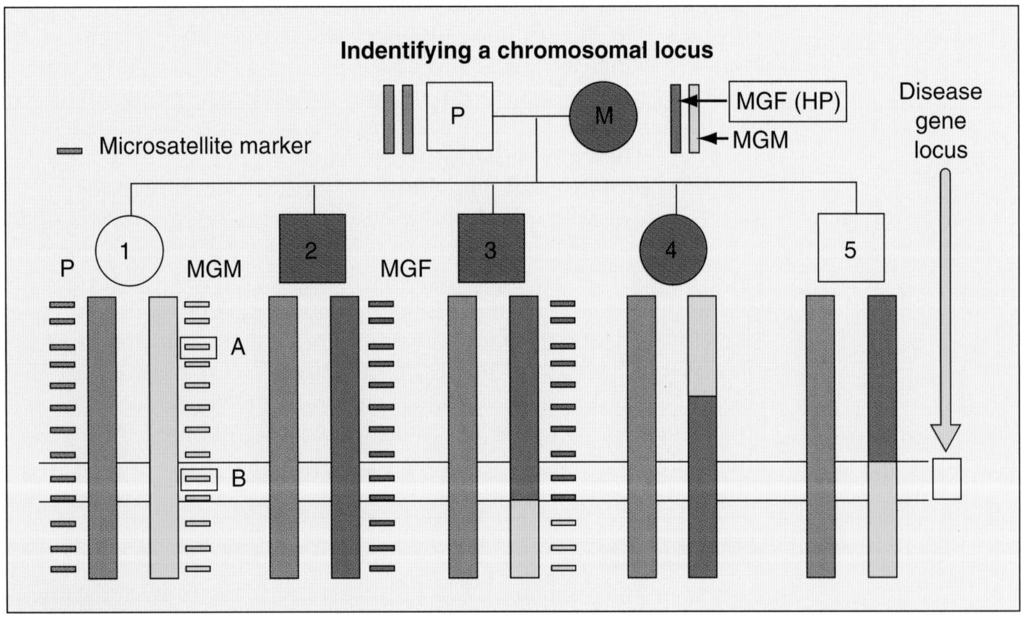

Indentifying a chromosomal locus

FIGURE 10-13.

Identification of a chromosomal locus. The affected mother (M) from Figure 10-12 is shown at the top. The homologous paternal chromosomes (P) are shown in gray. Hereditary pancreatitis was inherited by the mother from the maternal father (MGF, chromosome shown in red). The maternal grandmother (MGM, chromosome shown in yellow) does not have hereditary pancreatitis, and has a normal copy of the gene. Child #1, #2, #3, #4, and #5 are illustrated, with the three affected children highlighted in green. Microsatellite markers are indicated as short lines next to the chromosome below each child. By checking the microsatellite markers along this chromosome (child #1, far left), it can be determined that the entire maternal chromosome was inherited from the MGM; therefore, this appears in yellow. As expected, child #1 does not have pancreatitis. In child #2, the affected child inherited a complete copy of the maternal grandfather's chromosome and also inherited the disease. This chromosome from child #3 reveals that a crossover event occurred during meiosis. By looking at the microsatellite markers, we can determine that the last three markers were inherited from the MGM, who did not have the disease. Ten of the markers, however, were inherited from the MGM along with the disease; therefore, we know that the disease gene is somewhere above the yellow markers. Child #4 is a daughter who is affected with hereditary pancreatitis. Again, the microsatellite markers tell us that the top of the chromosome was inherited from the MGM, and therefore could not transmit the disease gene. Child #5 is a son who is not affected. In this case, most of the chromosome was inherited from the affected MGM, with only a portion of the chromosome inherited from the MGM. Therefore, by inference, the disease must be located within the small region shown to the far right. The inheritance of this disease is perfectly matched with microsatellite marker B, shown on the far left, but not with A. Therefore, by carefully plotting the inheritance of microsatellite markers through the family tree, the precise location of the disease gene can be determined.

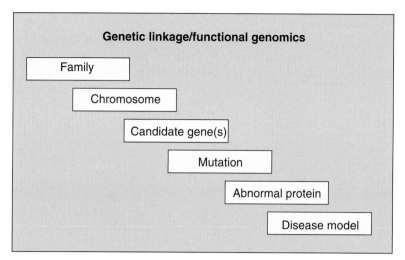

FIGURE 10-14.

Using this functional genomics approach, once a family has been identified, the chromosome locus is identified as illustrated in Figure 10-13, followed by a survey of candidate genes within this small region of the affected chromosome. The searches continue to narrow its focus until the mutation has been found and the consequences determined.

HEREDITARY PANCREATITIS GENE AND THE PATHOPHYSIOLOGIC MECHANISMS LEADING TO ACUTE AND CHRONIC PANCREATITIS

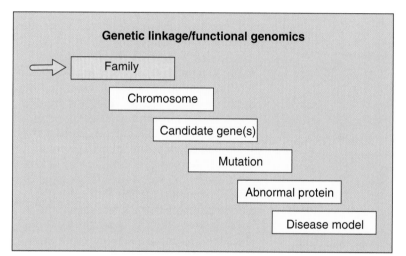

FIGURE 10-15.

The first step in discovering the cause of hereditary pancreatitis was to define a family appropriate to the study.

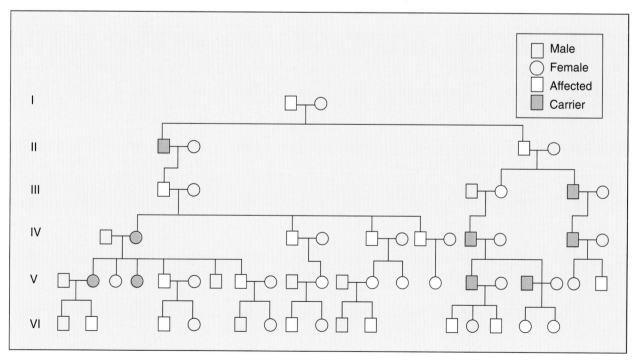

FIGURE 10-16.

Partial pedigree of the S-family used to map the hereditary pancreatitis gene [4]. This portion covers seven generations, from which individuals were chosen to optimize the mapping process. Family members with characteristic pancreatitis are shown in the solid symbols in white. Clinically unaffected individuals who carried the hereditary pancreatitis disease gene are shown in light blue. For the entire family, 80% of the individuals with the gene had clinical symptoms similar to those reported in other large families.

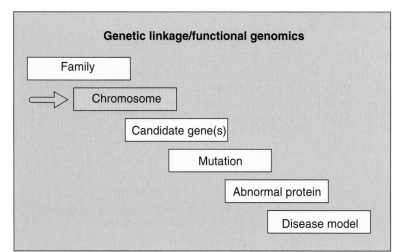

FIGURE 10-17.

The second step in discovering the cause of heredity pancreatitis was to establish linkage between hereditary pancreatitis and a specific region on a single chromosome segment.

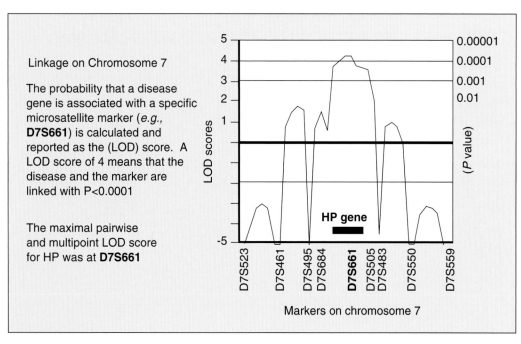

Linkage on Chromosome 7

The probability that a disease gene is associated with a specific microsatellite marker (*e.g.*, **D7S661**) is calculated and reported as the (LOD) score. A LOD score of 4 means that the disease and the marker are linked with P<0.0001

The maximal pairwise and multipoint LOD score for HP was at **D7S661**

HP gene

Markers on chromosome 7

FIGURE 10-18.

Linkage of hereditary pancreatitis to chromosome 7q35. To find the chromosome region containing the affected gene, microsatellite markers from a number of chromosomes were sequentially tested for linkage with the disease gene. This led to the identification of the

hereditary pancreatitis locus on chromosome 7 [4,7].

This figure illustrates the log of differences (LOD) score plot of microsatellite markers along chromosome 7 [4]. The X axis represents a portion of chromosome 7, with the short arm of the chromosome to the left and the long arm to the right. The code numbers (*eg*, D7S523, D7S461, etc) denote specific microsatellite markers and their approximate distance from each other. The Y axis on the left is the LOD score. The LOD score is a logarithmic probability scale. For example, an LOD score of 2 means that the probability that the inheritance of a microsatellite marker is randomly associated with the inheritance of the disease gene by chance is 1 in 100 (*eg*, P = 0.01). An LOD score of 4 means that the probability is 1:10,000 (P = 0.0001). Approximate P values are shown on the right. From these data, the LOD score from microsatellite D7S661 was 4.3. This was strong evidence that the hereditary pancreatitis gene was near this microsatellite marker. (*Adapted from* Whitcomb *et al.* [4].)

Identification of HP locus

Maximum multipoint LOD score at D7S661

D7S661 near the T-cell receptor β gene (TCRβ)

TCRβ known to be on 7q35

	7p	Chromosome 7
D7S517	6	
D7S507	29	
D7S516	45	
D7S528	62	
D7S521	67	
D7S691	68	
D7S506	77	
		Centromere
D7S524	105	
D7S523	134	
D7S461	147	
D7S495	159	
D7S684	163	
D7S661	171	HP gene
D7S505	177	
D7S483	182	
D7S550	196	
D7S559	203	
	7q	

FIGURE 10-19.

The region of chromosome 7, within which the hereditary pancreatitis gene was found to lie. Location of the hereditary pancreatitis gene is given in relation to the genetic map with the microsatellite markers shown on the left. Because of the large size of the family (over 500 members), it was possible to narrow the locus to within 19 centimorgans (green vertical bar), and thus to determine that it was within 7q35. (*Adapted from* Whitcomb *et al.* [4] and Le Bodic *et al.* [7].)

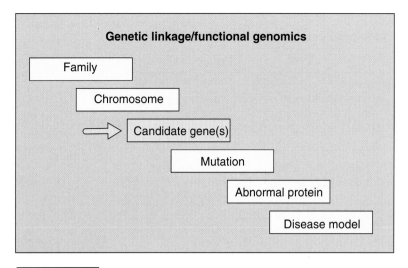

Genetic linkage/functional genomics

Family → Chromosome → Candidate gene(s) → Mutation → Abnormal protein → Disease model

FIGURE 10-20.

Having narrowed down the gene's location to this chromosome segment, candidate genes within that region could be identified.

TABLE 10-6. HEREDITARY PANCREATITIS: CANDIDATE GENES

Expression in the pancreas

Potential for activating digestive enzymes [8]

Exclusion of carboxypeptidase A1

Presence of 5 trypsinogen genes in the TCR-β complex [9]

Trypsinogen considered as the primary candidate gene

TABLE 10-6.

There were two key features that were believed to be important in selecting the primary candidate genes for mutational screening [3]. First, the gene should be expressed in the pancreas; second, it should have the potential of activating digestive enzymes [8]. Although carboxypeptidase A1 was an attractive candidate, it was outside the 7q35 region.

As part of the Human Genome Project, the entire 685,000 base TCR-β locus was sequenced and deposited into a genetic code database (GeneBank) early in 1996 [9]. Eight trypsinogen-like genes were identified within this sequence, three of which were pseudogenes. Two of the remaining five trypsinogen genes were identified as cationic trypsinogen and anionic trypsinogen, which were known to be expressed in high abundance in the pancreas. Therefore, the trypsinogens were considered the primary candidate genes.

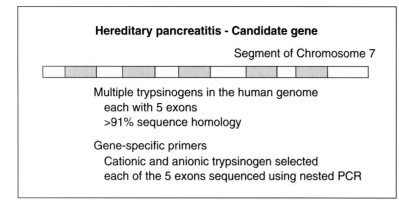

FIGURE 10-21.

The next problem is that each trypsinogen gene is very similar to the other trypsinogen genes. Each has five exons and greater than 91% sequence homology [8]. Therefore, amplifying any one gene by polymerase chain reaction (PCR) for DNA sequencing would likely result in cross-amplification from the other trypsin genes, and thus make identification of a single-point mutation in one of the two chromosomes almost impossible. To solve this problem, gene-specific primers were designed using a nested PCR strategy [3]. Each of the five exons from cationic and anionic trypsinogen could then be amplified and sequenced.

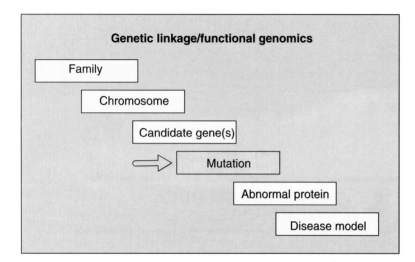

FIGURE 10-22.

Candidate genes are ready to be screened for mutations.

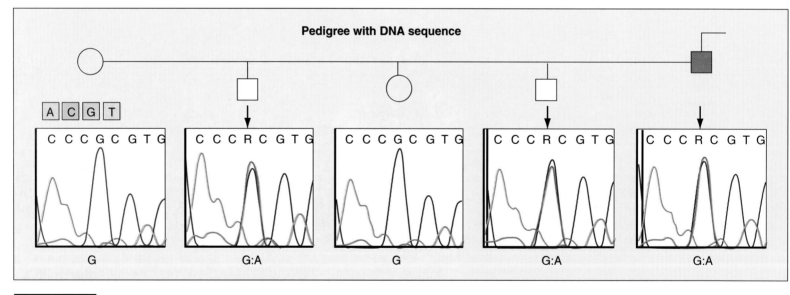

FIGURE 10-23.

On the top of this figure is a partial pedigree of one of the hereditary pancreatitis kindreds [3]. On the bottom is the DNA sequencing electropherograms aligned with the pedigree and showing the DNA sequence of the human cationic trypsinogen gene in the region of the hereditary pancreatitis mutation. Specimens from affected family members and obligate carrier members demonstrate heterozygosity at the fourth nucleotide in the frame (see arrows in the 2nd, 4th, and 5th panels). The sequencing signal is almost exactly 50% guanine (G) and 50% adenine (A) from each of these three specimens. In contrast, the signal observed for the two unaffected family members is 100% G at this site. Thus, the hereditary pancreatitis mutation was identified as a G-to-A mutation. This mutation is predicted to result in an arginine (R) to histidine (H) substitution at amino acid 117 of trypsin using the more common chymotrypsin numbering system (R117H).

TABLE 10-7. HEREDITARY PANCREATITIS: RESULTS

Single G:A transition mutation in the third exon of cation trypsinogen

S-family—mutation present in all affected members and obligate carriers

Four confirmatory families (3 from the United States, 1 from Italy): mutation present on all affected members and obligate carriers

Mutation absent in 16 unaffected obligates

TABLE 10-7.

A single guanine-to-adenine (G:A) mutation in the third exon of cationic trypsinogen was found in all affected and obligate carrier members of the S family [3]. This mutation was also found in all affected and obligate carriers in four confirmatory families. This mutation was not found in people who married into the family, and were therefore obligate unaffected family members [3].

G:A mutation creates a novel restriction site for *Afl* III.

Afl III digestion cut all the PCR products from exon 3 of all affected individuals and obligate carriers (**A**).

Afl III digestion cut none of the PCR products from obligate unaffected family members (**B**).

Afl III digestion cut none of the PCR products from 140 unrelated control individuals (**C**).

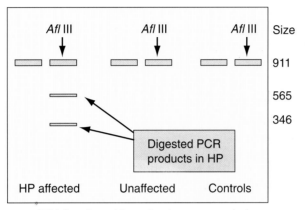

Ethidium bromide-stained agarose gel of PCR-amplified exon 3 products from the human cationic trypsinogen gene

FIGURE 10-24.

Guanine-to-adenine (G:A) mutation. Some variations in the DNA sequence represent harmless polymorphisms that are common in the general population. To determine if the G:A mutation was a natural polymorphism, a rapid screening assay has been developed (patent pending) [3]. The G:A mutation created a novel restriction enzyme cut site

for *Afl* III. Therefore, the DNA from individuals with hereditary pancreatitis would be digested by *Afl* III at the mutation site.

This figure illustrates *Afl* III digestion of the polymerase chain reaction (PCR)–amplified exon 3 products from the human cationic trypsinogen gene after separation on an agarose gel. The patient in A was affected with hereditary pancreatitis. The first lane contains the 911 base-pair (bp) product of PCR amplification that is undigested. Lane 2 is the same PCR product after *Afl* III digestion. Note that half the PCR product has been digested and migrates in the gel as 565 bp and 346 bp products. Using this screening method, all PCR products of all affected individuals and obligate carriers were digested by *Afl* III. The patients in B and C represent obligate unaffected and unrelated control DNA. *Afl* III failed to digest the PCR products from these individuals. Using this screening test, obligate carriers and 140 controls were shown to be without the R117H mutation.

FIGURE 10-25.

Having found the mutation, the consequence of the mutation can be determined. In the case of hereditary pancreatitis, the mutation changes a key amino acid into a protein.

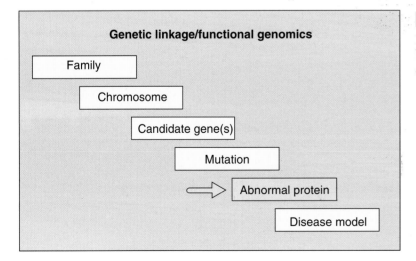

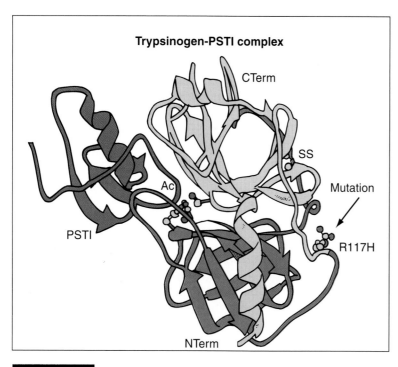

Trypsinogen-PSTI complex

FIGURE 10-26.

Ribbon diagram for the trypsinogen–trypsinogen inhibitor complex. The trypsinogen protein has two globular domains, shown in yellow and blue. These two globular domains are connected by a single peptide chain shown on the right side of the molecule. The active site of the trypsin enzyme is in a cleft on the opposite side of the molecule from the connecting chain. The pancreatic secretory trypsin inhibitor is shown as it fits into the specificity pocket and blocks the active sites.

The R117H mutation is in the middle of the connecting chain on the far right. This site is away from the trypsin activation site (behind the molecule, not shown) and is on the surface of the molecule opposite of the active site. Thus, it is unlikely that this mutation activates trypsin or changes its enzymatic function; however, biochemical studies have shown that arginine is the recognition site for trypsin-like enzymes and that R117 is the initial hydrolysis site in the trypsin degradation process. From this illustration, it is evident how severing the connection chain between the two globular domains can lead to permanent destruction of the enzyme as the active site is split. The R117H substitution removes the trypsin recognition site from the connecting chain and prevents hydrolysis at this site. Thus, the mutant trypsin is resistant to hydrolysis. (*Adapted from* Whitcomb [4]; with permission.)

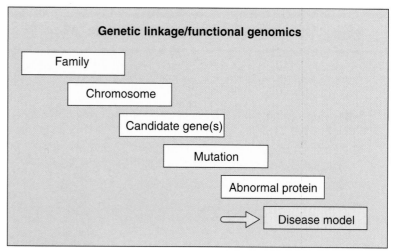

Genetic linkage/functional genomics

FIGURE 10-27.

The next step is to construct a model of the disease incorporating insights into the function or lack thereof in the abnormal gene. These disease models are important because they give insight into how therapeutic agents may be used to circumvent the problems arising from altered gene products.

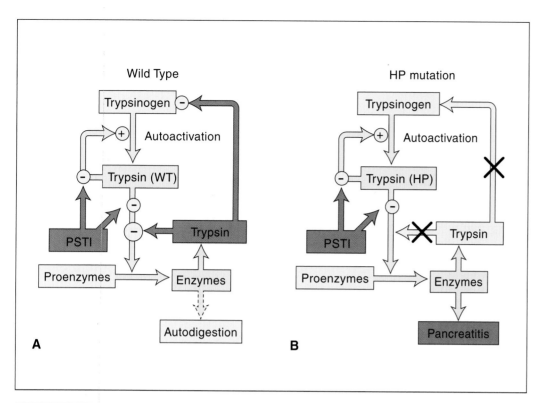

FIGURE 10-28.

A, The normal "wild-type" trypsinogen [3]. **B,** Effect of the mutation caused by hereditary pancreatitis. Within the normal pancreas (**panel A**) a fraction of the human trypsinogen autoactivates to trypsin. Trypsin, shown in yellow, has the potential of catalyzing a cascade of trypsinogen activation (above) and activation of all other proenzymes (below), leading to pancreatic autodigestion and pancreatitis; however, two control mechanisms exist that prevent this from happening within the pancreas. The first defense is pancreatic sectetory trypsin inhibitor (PSTI), shown in the red box on the left. PSTI is synthesized with

trypsinogen in a ratio of about 1:20. When levels of trypsin activity are low, PSTI quickly inhibits trypsin and prevents further autoactivation of trypsin and other proenzymes inside the pancreas; however, far more trypsinogen exists than PSTI. Therefore, during times of excessive trypsinogen activation, the inhibitory capacity of PSTI is overwhelmed; trypsin's activity continues to increase. Fortunately, a fail-safe mechanism is present to prevent uncontrolled enzyme activation and autodigestion. Under these circumstances, trypsin and trypsin-like enzymes feed back to hydrolyze the chain connecting the two globular domains of the trypsin at R117, resulting in permanent inactivation of trypsin and stopping the activation cascade. In this way, the healthy pancreas is protected from autodigestion.

Consider the model shown **panel B**. In patients who have the hereditary pancreatitis mutation, trypsinogen is autoactivated to trypsin as shown in the previous model. PSTI continues to function in a normal way, thus preventing trypsin from activating trypsinogen and all other pancreatic proenzymes; however, under conditions of excessive trypsinogen activation and those in which the inhibitory capacity of PSTI is overwhelmed, the R117 trypsin recognition is mutated, and therefore trypsin cannot be inactivated. "Super-trypsin" continues to drive the zymogen activation cascade, leading to autodigestion and pancreatitis.

TABLE 10-8. HEREDITARY PANCREATITIS: PROPOSED MECHANISM

Autosomal dominant requires that only half of trypsin molecules need to be resistant to hydrolysis

Intermittent attacks only occur when a greater amount of trypsin is present than can be inhibited by PSTI

TABLE 10-8.

This proposed mechanism explains why hereditary pancreatitis is an autosomal dominant disorder. Only half the trypsin molecules need to be resistant to hydrolysis to express the phenotype of autodigestion in pancreatitis. Second, it explains why attacks of pancreatitis are intermittent. In this model, attacks will only occur when more trypsin is active and can be inhibited by pancreatic secretary trypsin inhibitor. Thus, the model explains the key features of hereditary pancreatitis.

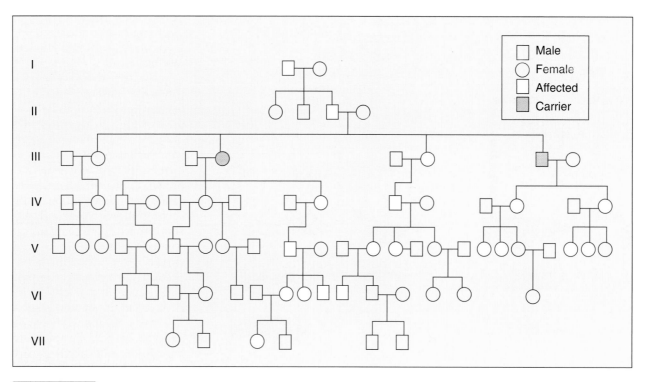

FIGURE 10-29.

Within 6 months of the report of the R117H mutation, many families with numerous hereditary pancreatitis throughout the United States, England, France, Italy, Germany, and Japan were identified with the same mutation; however, occasional families were noted that did not have this common mutation [10]. One of these families, initially described in 1967 by Robechek (R-family) [11], had over 60 family members and participated in a new genetic linkage study. Thirty members were interviewed, a family tree constructed, blood samples were obtained for linkage study, and the clinical characteristics were reviewed and compared with the S-family.

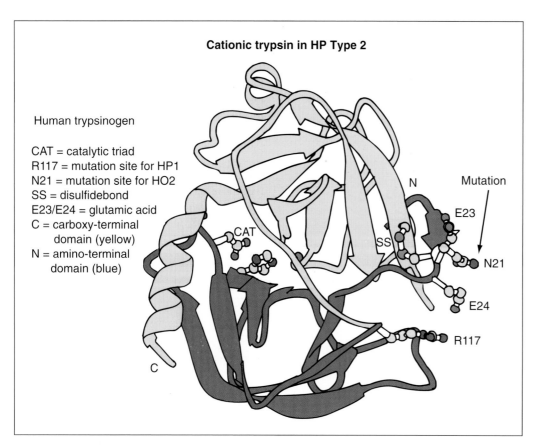

Cationic trypsin in HP Type 2

Human trypsinogen

CAT = catalytic triad
R117 = mutation site for HP1
N21 = mutation site for HO2
SS = disulfidebond
E23/E24 = glutamic acid
C = carboxy-terminal
      domain (yellow)
N = amino-terminal
      domain (blue)

FIGURE 10-30.

Linkage analysis proved that the disease gene is in chromosome 7, as seen in hereditary pancreatitis type 1. A mutation was identified in the cationic trypsinogen gene in all affected individuals. However, in hereditary pancreatitis type 2 the mutation was an asparagine-to-isoleucine substitution at position 21 (N21I) [10]. Identification of a second major mutation in the same cationic trypsinogen gene in a family with distinct clinical features of hereditary pancreatitis suggests that this molecule may play a critical role in the pathogenesis of acute pancreatitis in humans through inappropriate activation of digestive enzymes.

TABLE 10-9. HEREDITARY PANCREATITIS: CONCLUSIONS

A genome-wide search using genetic linkage analysis identified the hereditary pancreatitis gene on chromosome 7

An R117H mutation in the cationic trypsinogen gene occurs in most of the studied families with hereditary pancreatitis

Molecular modeling predicts formation of hydrolysis-resistant tryspsin that could lead to pancreatic autodigestion

Implications of these findings for both acute and chronic pancreatitis, as well as pancreatic cancer, have yet to be determined.

TABLE 10-9.

In summary, a genome-wide search using genetic linkage analysis identified hereditary pancreatitis on genome chromosome 7. An R117H or N21I mutation in the cationic trypsinogen gene occurs in most families with hereditary pancreatitis studied. Molecular modeling predicts formation of hydrolysis-resistant trypsin that could lead to pancreatic autodigestion.

TABLE 10-10. HEREDITARY PANCREATITIS: NEW INSIGHTS

Importance of premature trypsin activation

Chronic pancreatitis results from recurrent acute pancreatitis

Chronic inflammation strongly predisposes the patient to pancreatic cancer

Hereditary pancreatitis may prove to be an excellent "model" for the study of many aspects of pancreatitis and pancreatic cancer

TABLE 10-10.

The study of hereditary pancreatitis has resulted in some new important insights into diseases of the pancreas. First, it demonstrates for the first time the importance of premature trypsin activation in the development of acute pancreatitis. Second, it provides direct evidence that chronic pancreatitis results from recurrent acute pancreatitis. Third, it emphasizes the importance of chronic pancreatic inflammation in the development of pancreatic cancer. Finally, hereditary pancreatitis may be an excellent human model for studying many aspects of acute and chronic pancreatitis, as well as pancreatic cancer.

ACKNOWLEDGMENTS

The author would like to thank Dr. William Furrey for x-ray crystallography images, Charles Ulrich II, MD for reviewing the presentation, and Julia LaSalle for editorial assistance.

REFERENCES

1. Perrault J: Hereditary pancreatitis. *Gastroenterol Clin North Am* 1994, 23:743–752.

2. Comfort M, Steinberg A: Pedigree of a family with hereditary chronic relapsing pancreatitis. *Gastroenterology* 1952, 21:54–63.

3. Whitcomb DC, Gorry MC, Preston RA, *et al.*:Hereditary pancreatitis is caused by a mutation in the cationic trypsinogen gene. *Nat Genet* 1996, 14:141–145.

4. Whitcomb DC, Preston RA, Aston CE, *et al.*: A gene for hereditary pancreatitis maps to chromosome 7q35. *Gastroenterology* 1996, 110:1975–1980.

5. Kattwinkel J, Lapey A, Di SAP, Edwards WA: Hereditary pancreatitis: Three new kindreds and a critical review of the literature. *Pediatrics* 1973, 51:55–69.

6. Collins FS: Molecular genetics in clinical practice I: Sequencing the human genome. *Hosp Pract* 1997, 32:35–53.

7. Le Bodic L, Bignon JD, Raguenes O, *et al.*: The hereditary pancreatitis gene maps to long arm of chromosome 7. *Hum Mol Genet* 1996, 5:549–554.

8. Chiari H: Ueber selbstverdauung des menschlichen pankreas. Zeitschrift fur Heilkunde 1896, 17:69–96.

9. Rowen L, Koop BF, Hood L: The complete 685-kilobase DNA sequence of the human beta T cell receptor locus. *Science* 1996, 272:1755–1762.

10. Gorry M, Gabbaizedeh D, Furey W, *et al.*: Multiple mutations in the cationic trypsinogen gene are associated with hereditary pancreatitis. *Gastroenterology* 1997, in press.

11. Robechek PJ: Hereditary chronic relapsing pancreatitis: A clue to pancreatitis in general? *Am J Surg* 1967, 113:819–824.

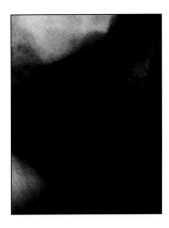

Index

Page numbers followed by *t* or *f* indicate tables or figures, respectively.

D

Duodenal diverticula, periampullary, acute pancreatitis caused by, 3.2*t*
Duodenum
cholecystokinin release, feedback inhibition of, 1.11–1.12
in pancreatic control system, 1.3*f*, 1.5*f*

E

Ectopic pancreas, 6.12*t*
Elastase
in chronic pancreatitis, 4.13*f*
fecal, in diagnosis of chronic pancreatitis, 4.9*f*
Endoscopic retrograde cholangiopancreatography
acinarization of pancreas during, 6.6*f*
acute pancreatitis caused by, 3.4*t*
in chronic pancreatitis, 4.18*f*, 5.5*t*, 5.9*f*, 5.10*f*–5.11*f*
emergency, in acute pancreatitis, 3.11
in gallstone pancreatitis, 3.1–3.2
in idiopathic acute pancreatitis, 3.4*t*, 6.18*t*
in pancreatic cancer, 7.13*f*, 7.13*t*, 7.14*f*
diagnostic, 7.2, 7.5*f*
findings, 7.10*f*
Endoscopic retrograde pancreatography
in diagnosis of chronic pancreatitis, 4.6*f*, 4.6*t*, 4.7*f*, 4.8*t*
in pancreas divisum, 4.7*f*
Endoscopic sphincterotomy, in management of acute pancreatitis, 3.11*t*
Endoscopy
in pancreatic cancer, 7.13–7.14
therapeutic, for pain relief, in chronic pancreatitis, 4.16*f*
Energy deficit, in cystic fibrosis, pathogenesis of, 9.18*f*
Energy imbalance, in cystic fibrosis
causes of, 9.17*f*
pathogenesis of, 9.17*f*
Enkephalin, and pancreatic secretion, 1.14*t*
Epidermal growth factor, clinical applications, 8.5*t*
Epithelial cell transport, 9.3*f*
ERCP. *See* Endoscopic retrograde cholangiopancreatography
ERP. *See* Endoscopic retrograde pancreatography
Esophageal reflux, in cystic fibrosis, 9.9*t*, 9.10*f*
Estrogens, acute pancreatitis caused by, 3.3*t*
Ethanol. *See* Alcohol

F

Fat necrosis, with acute pancreatitis, 3.6*f*
Fecal fat. *See also* Steatorrhea
staining for
in chronic pancreatitis, 4.17*f*
in cystic fibrosis, 9.13*f*
Feedback control mechanisms
in cholecystokinin release, 1.11–1.12
in pancreatic control system, 1.5*f*
sensation and amplification for, 1.5*f*
Fibroblast growth factor, receptors, in pancreatic cancer, 2.7*t*
5-Fluorouracil, for pancreatic cancer, 7.19*t*
Foreign body, pancreatic duct obstruction by, acute pancreatitis caused by, 3.2*t*

Functional genomics
definition of, 10.5*f*
in hereditary pancreatitis, 10.5*f*, 10.6*f*, 10.9*f*–10.14*f*
Fungi, acute pancreatitis caused by, 3.3*t*

G

Gabexate, effects on mortality in acute pancreatitis, 2.3*f*
Gallbladder, radioligand imaging of, 8.7*f*
Gallstones, acute pancreatitis caused by, 3.1, 3.2*t*, 3.5*f*
endoscopic retrograde cholangiopancreatography in, 3.11*t*
Ranson criteria for severity of, 3.7*t*, 3.8*t*
Gastrinoma
clinical applications of peptide and peptide analogues in, 8.5*t*
radioligand imaging of, 8.8*f*
somatostatin analogue and, 8.4*t*
Gastrin-releasing peptide
clinical applications, 8.5*t*
and pancreas, 1.4*f*
Gastroesophageal reflux, in cystic fibrosis, 9.9*t*, 9.10*f*
Gastrointestinal tract, in pancreatic control system, 1.3*f*
Gene mapping, 10.7*f*
Genetic linkage analysis, in hereditary pancreatitis, 10.1, 10.5*f*, 10.5*t*, 10.9*f*–10.14*f*, 10.16*f*
Genetic recombination, in meiosis, 10.6*f*
Genetics
of cystic fibrosis, 9.1, 9.2–9.4
of hereditary pancreatitis, 10.1
of pancreatic cancer, 2.7*t*
Genetic studies, 10.6–10.9
GHRFoma, somatostatin analogue and, 8.4*t*
Glasgow score, for severity of acute pancreatitis, 3.7*t*
Glioma, clinical applications of peptide and peptide analogues in, 8.5*t*
Glucagon
and pancreatic secretion, 1.14*t*
secretion, 1.3*f*
Glucagonoma
radioligand imaging of, 8.11*f*
somatostatin analogue and, 8.4*t*
Glycoprotein(s)
CD44, gene mutations, in pancreatic cancer, 2.7*t*
GP-2, in chronic pancreatitis, 2.6*t*
Growth hormone-producing tumor, somatostatin analogue and, 8.4*t*

H

Head of pancreas, spiral (loop) contour in, 6.15*f*
Hereditary pancreatitis, 3.2*t*, 3.3*t*, 4.3*f*, 5.2, 5.4*t*, 10.1–10.17
candidate genes, 10.11*f*, 10.11*t*, 10.12*f*
clinical findings in, 10.2*t*, 10.3*f*
definition of, 10.2*t*
disease model, 10.14*f*, 10.15*f*, 10.15*t*
epidemiology of, 10.1, 10.4*f*
etiology of, 10.1, 10.4–10.6
identification of, by traditional methods, 10.4*t*
proposed, 10.4*t*
functional genomics in, 10.5*f*, 10.6*f*, 10.9*f*–10.14*f*
gene, 10.1, 10.9–10.17
genetic linkage analysis in, 10.1, 10.5*f*, 10.5*t*, 10.9*f*–10.14*f*, 10.16*f*
genetics of, 10.1